# Substance Abusing Latinos: Current Research on Epidemiology, Prevention, and Treatment

*Substance Abusing Latinos: Current Research on Epidemiology, Prevention, and Treatment* has been co-published simultaneously as *Journal of Social Work Practice in the Addictions*, Volume 5, Numbers 1/2 2005.

**Monographic Separates from the *Journal of Social Work Practice in the Addictions***

For additional information on these and other Haworth Press titles, including descriptions, tables of contents, reviews, and prices, use the QuickSearch catalog at http://www.HaworthPress.com.

***Substance Abusing Latinos: Current Research on Epidemiology, Prevention, and Treatment,*** edited by Mario R. De La Rosa, PhD, Lori K. Holleran, PhD, Shulamith Lala Ashenberg Straussner, DSW, CAS (Vol. 5, No. 1/2, 2005). *Examines the latest information, research, and recent advances in the prevention of substance abuse and HIV/AIDS in Latino populations.*

***International Aspects of Social Work Practice in the Addictions,*** edited by Shulamith Lala Ashenberg Straussner, DSW, CAS, and Larry Harrison, MA, CQSW (Vol. 2, No. 3/4, 2002). *"Provides valuable insight into one of the most significant changes in social life during the last fifty years and indicates some of the likely direction for changes in the first half of the twenty-first century." (Tony Clamp, DipCouns, DipSW, MA, Lecturer in Applied Social Studies, University of Durham, United Kingdom)*

***Neurobiology of Addictions: Implications for Clinical Practice,*** edited by Richard T. Spence, PhD, MSSW, Diana M. DiNitto, PhD, and Shulamith Lala Ashenberg Straussner, DSW, CAS (Vol. 1, No. 3, 2001). *Presents the neurobiological theories of addiction in a psychosocial context and connects the theoretical information with practical applications.*

# Substance Abusing Latinos: Current Research on Epidemiology, Prevention, and Treatment

Mario R. De La Rosa
Lori K. Holleran
Shulamith Lala Ashenberg Straussner
Editors

*Substance Abusing Latinos: Current Research on Epidemiology, Prevention, and Treatment* has been co-published simultaneously as *Journal of Social Work Practice in the Addictions,* Volume 5, Numbers 1/2 2005.

Routledge
Taylor & Francis Group
LONDON AND NEW YORK

Published by

The Haworth Social Work Practice Press, 10 Alice Street, Binghamton, NY 13904-1580 USA

Published 2017 by Routledge

711 Third Avenue, New York, NY, 100017

2 Park Square, Milton Park, Abingdon, Oxon, OX14 4RN

*Substance Abusing Latinos: Current Research on Epidemiology, Prevention, and Treatment* has been co-published simultaneously as *Journal of Social Work Practice in the Addictions*, Volume 5, Numbers 1/2 2005.



Cover design by Lora Wiggins

**Library of Congress Cataloging-in-Publication Data**

Substance abusing Latinos: current research on epidemiology, prevention, and treatment/Mario R. De La Rosa, Lori K. Holleran, Shulamith Lala Ashenberg Straussner, editors.
p. cm.
"Co-published simultaneously as Journal of social work practice in the addictions, volume 5, numbers 1/2 2005."
Includes bibliographical references and index.
ISBN-13: 978-07890-2882-2 (hc. : alk. paper)
ISBN-10: 0-7890-2882-4 (hc. : alk. paper)
ISBN-13: 978-07890-2883-9 (pbk. : alk. paper)
ISBN-10: 0-7890-2883-2 (pbk. : alk. paper)
1. Hispanic Americans–Substance use. 2. Hispanic Americans–Substance use–Prevention. 3. Substance abuse–United States–Prevention. I. De La Rosa, Mario R. II. Holleran, Lori K. III. Straussner, Shulamith Lala Ashenberg. IV. Journal of social work practice in the addictions.
HV5824.E85.S835 2005
362.29'089'68073-dc22 2004027877

# Substance Abusing Latinos: Current Research on Epidemiology, Prevention, and Treatment

## CONTENTS

## ABOUT THE EDITORS

**Mario B. De La Rosa, PhD,** is Associate Professor in the School of Social Work in the College of Health and Urban Affairs at Florida International University. Before joining FIU Dr. De La Rosa was Visiting Research Associate Professor at Boston University's School of Social Work, a Health Science Administrator with the National Institute on Drug Abuse (NIDA), and a Visiting Scholar at Harvard University's David Rockefeller Center for Latin America Studies. Dr. De La Rosa has published more than 50 scientific manuscripts on the etiology of drug use with Latino populations and related consequences. He is currently the principal investigator of two National Institutes of Health (NIH) funded research center grants. Dr. De La Rosa is the recipient of the 1996 American Association for the Advancement of Science award for outstanding work in the substance abuse field, and the 1989 Outstanding Alumni Award from the Office of Minority Affairs, the Ohio State University.

**Lori K. Holleran, PhD, ACSW,** is Assistant Professor in the School of Social Work at the University of Texas at Austin. Before joining UT, Dr. Holleran did clinical work in the area of addictions, supervised adolescent drug counselors, and worked as Research Associate and Ethnographic Analyst on a variety of projects including the Drug Resistance Strategies (DRS) Project. Dr. Holleran has done research in early intervention alcohol prevention and culturally grounded prevention interventions with Mexican Americans. She is currently working on her K01 Mentored Research Scientist Development grant funded by the National Institute on Drug Abuse in the area of culturally grounded substance abuse prevention with high-risk youth in community settings.

**Shulamith Lala Ashenberg Straussner, DSW, CEAP, BCD, CAS,** is Professor at New York University School of Social Work. She was a Fulbright Senior Scholar to Israel in 2003; Distinguished Visiting Professor, Ben Gurion University, Israel, in January 2002; and Visiting Professor, Omsk State Pedagogical University in Siberia, Russia, Spring, 2000.

Dr. Straussner has numerous publications dealing with substance abuse. Among her thirteen books are: *Clinical Work with Substance Abusing Clients* (Guilford Press, 1994/2004); *International Aspects of Social Work Practice in the Addictions* (co-edited with L. Harrison, The Haworth Press, Inc., 2003); *Understanding Mass Violence: A Social Work Perspective* (co-edited with Norma Phillips, Allyn & Bacon, 2003); *The Handbook of Addiction Treatment for Women* (co-edited with Stephanie Brown, Jossey-Bass, 2002); *Ethnocultural Factors in Addictions Treatment* (Guilford Press, 2001); and *Gender and Addictions: Men and Women in Treatment* (co-edited with E. Zelvin, Jason Aronson Press, 1997). She is the founding editor of the *Journal of Social Work Practice in the Addictions* (The Haworth Press, Inc.)

Dr. Straussner is Regional Director, Project MAINSTREAM, a HRSA/CSAT/AMERSA sponsored national project to expend interdisciplinary AOD training within 17 different health and mental health professions. She has served on the National Center on Substance Abuse Treatment and is a founding board member of the New York State Institute for Professional Development in Addictions. Dr. Straussner is the past chair of NASW Section on Alcohol, Tobacco, and Other Drugs. She received the Social Worker of the Year Award from the NASW ATOD Section in 2000 and Award for Individual Distinction in Addictions Education and Training from NY State IDPA in 2003.

Dr. Straussner serves as a consultant to various hospitals and other organizations and lectures on a variety of topics throughout the U.S. and abroad. She is trained in psychoanalytic psychotherapy, family, and group therapy and has a private therapeutic and supervisory practice in New York City.

∞ ALL HAWORTH SOCIAL WORK PRACTICE PRESS BOOKS AND JOURNALS ARE PRINTED ON CERTIFIED ACID-FREE PAPER

# Preface

During the past fifteen years there has been a concerted effort to understand the growing problem of substance abuse among Latino populations in the United States, yet information about the substance abuse behaviors of Latinos and the effectiveness of culturally relevant drug treatment and prevention services is still limited. Even more limited is information on the factors associated with substance abuse behaviors among vulnerable Latino subpopulations such as gang members, homeless women, and juvenile delinquent Latinos. What role does membership in gangs have on the onset of substance abuse among Latino gang members? What impact does childhood sexual abuse have on adult drug use among low-income urban Puerto Rican women? What relationship do acculturation and healthy family role models have with substance abuse behaviors of Cuban juvenile offenders?

Information on the effects that cultural, familial, and environmental factors have in the provision of effective drug prevention and treatment services to vulnerable Latino populations is similarly limited. Numerous poignant questions loom in this regard. What impact would the possibility of choosing provision of services in English or Spanish have on the effectiveness of substance abuse prevention services among Latino adolescents? How do parenting skills and their level of acculturation to the values and beliefs system of the United States affect the utilization of outpatient drug treatment counseling by substance abusing Latino adolescents? How does lack of health insurance, prior mental health care history, and involvement with the criminal justice system affect drug using Latino women's utilization of methadone maintenance program?

The purpose of this volume is to augment the extant literature on the extent and nature of substance abuse among vulnerable Latino subpop-

[Haworth co-indexing entry note]: "Preface." De La Rosa, Mario, R., Lori K. Holleran, and Shulamith Lala Ashenberg Straussner. Co-published simultaneously in *Journal of Social Work Practice in the Addictions* (The Haworth Press, Inc.) Vol. 5, No.1/2, 2005, pp. xxiii-xxvi; and: *Substance Abusing Latinos: Current Research on Epidemiology, Prevention, and Treatment* (ed: Mario R. De La Rosa, Lori K. Holleran, and Shulamith Lala Ashenberg Straussner) The Haworth Press, Inc., 2005, pp. xv-xviii. Single or multiple copies of this article are available for a fee from The Haworth Document Delivery Service [1-800-HAWORTH, 9:00 a.m. - 5:00 p.m. (EST). E-mail address: docdelivery@haworthpress.com].

http://www.haworthpress.com/web/JSWPA

ulations and to increase the knowledge base regarding the role that cultural, familial, and environmental factors have in the development of effective drug abuse interventions for these subpopulations. In this regard, the articles included in this special issue focus on providing information on the patterns of substance abuse among Latino gang members, Cuban juvenile offenders, and Puerto Rican homeless women. This volume also includes articles that discuss the role that acculturation factors, parenting skills, availability of insurance, and prior experience with mental health care and the justice system have on the provision of effective drug prevention and treatment services to vulnerable Latino populations.

The first article by De La Rosa, Holleran, Rugh, and MacMaster, provides a comprehensive review of research on the extent and nature of substance abuse among Latinos in the United States and the provision of culturally competent drug abuse prevention and treatment programs to Latino populations. The authors found that while significant progress has been made in understanding the drug using behaviors of Latinos and the importance of developing culturally competent substance abuse intervention programs, there are significant gaps in this area of research. The next article, by De La Rosa, Rugh, and Rojas, focuses on documenting the onset and progression of drug abuse in a cohort of Puerto Rican and Dominican gang members living in a small city. The findings from this research indicate, not surprisingly, that the onset of drug use among Latino gang members comes at a very early age and that progression to serious drug use occurs rapidly.

Vera, Alegría, Pattatucci-Aragón, and Peña's article examines the relationship between childhood sexual abuse and adult drug use among a cohort of drug using and non-using low-income urban Puerto Rican women. The results from this article provide further proof of the direct relationship between childhood sexual abuse and adult drug use found in other drug abusing populations. The article by Dévieux, Malow, Ergon-Pérez, Samuels, Rojas, Khushal, and Jean-Gilles examines the sexual and drug using behaviors of a much understudied vulnerable population: African American and Cuban American juvenile offenders. The results indicate that Cuban American adolescents showed higher levels of unprotected sex, higher levels of sex while using drugs, and higher levels of drug/alcohol use three and six months prior to confinement. These differences may be explained by multiple factors, including differences in acculturation levels among the Cuban

American adolescents, differences in health messages targeted at the two groups, and family mores and norms.

Culture, acculturation, and language are powerful issues in Latino/a research. The articles by Marsiglia, Kulis, Wagstaff, Elek, and Dran and by Crunkilton, Paz, and Boyle both focus on exploring the role that acculturation and Latino family beliefs and attitudes have in the effective delivery of prevention education services to Latino adolescents. The article by Marsiglia et al. addresses a major research gap in the literature: the role of language preference as a significant element in the provision of effective delivery of drug prevention services to Latino adolescents. This article's findings suggest that providing prevention education services in the language preferred by the Latino adolescents increases the effectiveness of the intervention in reducing or preventing their drug using behaviors. English speaking Latino adolescents showed the most favorable outcomes in reducing their drug using behaviors while Spanish speaking adolescents increased their negative attitudes toward the use of drugs. Similarly, Crunkilton, Paz, and Boyle's article also found that the incorporation of culturally appropriate language, beliefs, values, and principles improved the effectiveness of prevention programs providing substance abuse education to families. Both of these illustrated the importance of using a cultural approach in the provision of prevention education programs to Latino adolescents or their families.

Improving drug treatment utilization by drug using Latino adolescents and adult women is the purpose of the last two articles in this volume. Santisteban, Dillon, Mena, Estrada, and Vaughan focus on addressing the vexing problem of engaging Latino substance abusing parents and their families in drug treatment services. This study's findings indicate that Latino adolescents with lower levels of mental health disorders and parents with better parenting strategies were more likely to be engaged in drug treatment services than those who did not have such characteristics or conditions. Lundgren, Amaro, and Ben-Ami also examine drug treatment utilization by another vulnerable population: drug using Puerto Rican women. This article's findings suggest that lack of insurance, prior history of involvement with mental health services, and involvement with the justice system were the best predictors of drug treatment service utilization by Puerto Rican women.

In order to illuminate how the research topics and findings of this edition overlap with clients' and clinicians' experiences, this volume features two pieces that strike "where the rubber hits the road." A special topics interview by Holleran with Jennifer Herrera, Director of Prevention Programs for AIDS Services of Austin, in Texas, elucidates issues related to Latino/a clients, such as poverty, HIV/AIDS, mental health concerns, substance abuse problems, gender issues, and barriers to getting help. Outreach and intervention strategies are shared including peer educators, the use of "Platicas," and two evidence-based interventions: VOICES/VOCES behavioral change group and Reducing AIDS Risk Activities (RARA). The volume concludes with an autobiographical story of a bi-cultural Latina alcoholic and drug addict in recovery.

*Mario R. De La Rosa*
*Lori K. Holleran*
*Shulamith Lala Ashenberg Straussner*
*August, 2004*

# Substance Abuse Among U.S. Latinos: A Review of the Literature

Mario R. De La Rosa
Lori K. Holleran
Douglas Rugh
Samuel A. MacMaster

**SUMMARY.** Latinos have recently become the largest minority in the United States. High fertility and high immigration rates suggest continued high rate of growth. Alcohol and illicit drug use within this population give reason for concern. Beginning in early adolescence, Latinos and Native Americans lead the nation in alcohol and illicit drug use. They also have a high need for alcohol and illicit drug treatment compared to Whites and African-Americans. Research concerning ethnic differences is reviewed in order to gain an understanding of the patterns and trajectories of substance use within the Latino community. Prevention and treatment interventions specific to Latinos are described, and gaps in the literature are noted. Finally, implications of the current re-

---

Mario R. De La Rosa, PhD, is Associate Professor, Florida International University, School of Social Work, 11200 SW 8th Street, Miami, FL 33199 (E-mail: mario.de_la_rosa@fiu.edu). Lori K. Holleran, PhD, ACSW, is Assistant Professor, The University of Texas at Austin, School of Social Work, 1925 San Jacinto Boulevard, Austin, TX 78712-1203. Douglas Rugh, MSW, is Research Assistant and PhD candidate, Latino Drug Abuse Research Center, College of Health and Urban Affairs, Florida International University. Samuel A. MacMaster, PhD, is Assistant Professor, College of Social Work, University of Tennessee, 193 East Polk Avenue, Nashville, TN 37210.

[Haworth co-indexing entry note]: "Substance Abuse Among U.S. Latinos: A Review of the Literature." De La Rosa, Mario R. et al. Co-published simultaneously in *Journal of Social Work Practice in the Addictions* (The Haworth Press, Inc.) Vol. 5, No. 1/2, 2005, pp. 1-20; and: *Substance Abusing Latinos: Current Research on Epidemiology, Prevention, and Treatment* (ed: Mario R. De La Rosa, Lori K. Holleran, and Shulamith Lala Ashenberg Straussner) The Haworth Press, Inc., 2005, pp. 1-20. Single or multiple copies of this article are available for a fee from The Haworth Document Delivery Service [1-800-HAWORTH, 9:00 a.m. - 5:00 p.m. (EST). E-mail address: docdelivery@haworthpress.com].

http://www.haworthpress.com/web/JSWPA

Digital Object Identifier: 10.1300/J160v05n01_01

search findings for social workers and recommendations for future research are discussed. *[Article copies available for a fee from The Haworth Document Delivery Service: 1-800-HAWORTH. E-mail address: <docdelivery@haworthpress.com> Website: <http://www.HaworthPress.com>* 

**KEYWORDS.** Substance abuse, Latinos, literature review, treatment implications

## *INTRODUCTION*

Scientists have long recognized that individuals across different cultures and ethnicities manifest different drug using patterns, trajectories, and consequences associated with such use. Even though family and peers have been shown to play an important role in the etiology of substance abuse across ethnic groups (Brook, Whiteman, Balka, & Cohen, 1997; Epstein, Williams, & Botvin, 2002), research also indicates that important differences exist within ethnic groups on these and other factors.[1] This article highlights the research that demonstrates these differences in relation to the Latino population.[2]

The manuscript is organized along the following six dimensions: (1) a discussion of the U.S. Latino population geographic distribution, demographic characteristics, and socio-economic status; (2) the prevalence of substance use among Latinos and the consequences associated with such use; (3) a review of the underlying individual, familial, peer group, cultural, and communal factors associated with the substance abuse behaviors of Latinos; (4) a critical analysis of the research advances made in developing drug prevention education and treatments programs to address the specific needs of Latino populations; (5) a discussion on the role of the social work profession in addressing the growing problem of substance abuse in Latino populations; and (6) recommendations for future research.

## *THE U.S. LATINO POPULATION*

Data from the 2000 U.S Census indicates that 35.5 million Latinos or 12% of the U.S population live in the United States. The 2000 U.S Census also indicates that during the 1990s, the Latino population increased by 58%, from 22.4 million in 1990 to 35.3 million. This is five times more rapidly than any other ethnic group (Guzman, 2001). According to census data, people of Mexican descent comprise the largest Latino population subgroup, followed by persons of South and Central American descent. Furthermore, the census shows that during the last decade there was a 97% increase in immigrants from South and Central American countries.

About three quarters of all Latinos live in four states: Florida, California, New York, and Texas (Guzman, 2001). Almost 40% of the Latino population is foreign-born, and 35% are under the age of 18 (Schmidley, 2001). Additionally, Latinos have disproportionately low incomes (23% have income below the poverty line) and low levels of educational attainment (Therrien & Ramirez, 2000).

Despite the diverse nature of the Latino population in the United States, research exploring social, economic, and health variables of Latinos has not accounted for between-group and within-group differences among the various Latino population subgroups (Gloria & Peregoy, 1996; Trimble, 1995). Thus, research findings on Latinos may be misleading and given to overgeneralizations to all Latino subgroups when data from many of the studies included in their sample individuals of mostly Mexican and Puerto Rican origin (Straussner, 2001).

## *THE PREVALENCE OF SUBSTANCE ABUSE AMONG U.S. LATINOS*

Research studies have documented serious substance-using problems among various Latinos populations. During the past twenty years, efforts have been made to collect information on the prevalence of substance abuse in Latino populations. Emerging from this research are the following findings:

- The lifetime substance-use rates for Latinos are between the higher rates of European Americans and the lower rates of African Americans (Beauvais & Oetting, 2002).
- Data from the combined 2000 and 2001 National Household Survey of Drug Abuse[3] (NSDUH) show that rates of past-month illicit drug use in the Latino population (aged 12 or older) ranged from 9.2% for Puerto Ricans to 3.6% for Central or South Americans.
- Data from the Monitoring the Future (MTF), a school based survey, indicates that Cuban adolescents have the highest reported

12-month illicit drug-use rates of any ethnic group in the U.S. (Wallace, Bachman, O'Malley, Johnston, Schulenberg & Cooper, 2002).[4]

- Trend data from the MTF reveals that during the past decade, Latino youth 8th grade (12 to 13 years old) begin to display elevated prevalence rates for alcohol, marijuana, cocaine, heroin, tranquilizers, MDMA (ecstasy), and LSD (a national sample of students probabilistically drawn from public and private schools. The sample is intended to provide an unbiased representation of school students throughout the coterminous United States. Multistage area probability sample design involving three selection stages: (1) geographic areas or primary sampling units (PSUs), (2) schools (or linked groups of schools) within PSUs, and (3) students within sampled schools. The sample for the 2002 survey consists of approximately 16,000 students within 133 schools.
- Consequently, Latinos have the highest rate of substance use for that age group in the nation. However, data from the MTF also indicate that after the 8th grade, the prevalence rates of substance abuse among Latinos is comparable to that of whites.
- Data from the NSDUH indicates that among persons 12 years or older in 2001, the rates for illicit drug and alcohol dependence or abuse were 7.8% among Latinos, 7.5% among whites, and 6.2% among African-Americans.
- Data from the NSDUH indicates that in 2001, 3.3 percent of Latinos needed treatment for illicit drug problems compared to 3.1 percent of African-Americans and 2.6 percent of whites.
- Prevalence data indicate the rate of drug use among Latino females has historically been significantly lower than that of Latino males (Anthony, Warner, & Kessler, 1994; Hughes, Day, Marcantonio, & Torpy, 1997). Latina women also report lower rates of substance use compared to non-Latina white women (Young & Harrison, 2001).
- Research by Valdez (2000) suggests that although substance use may be lower among Latina women, the rates of abuse and dependence, once drug use has begun, may not differ.
- Recent studies indicate a troubling trend in which Latinas are using at rates similar to Latinos (Warner, Canino, & Colon, 2001), and in some instances higher rates have been reported for females (Kandel, Chen, Warner, Kessler, & Grant, 1997; Sloboda, 2002).

Overall, research on the drug using behaviors of Latino populations indicates that Latinos have high prevalence rates for substance abuse, the highest reported symptoms of dependency, and they have the highest need for alcohol and drug treatment compared to Whites and African-Americans. Findings from this research also show wide variations in the prevalence of drug use among the various Latino subpopulations, including gender.

## *CONSEQUENCES ASSOCIATED WITH SUBSTANCE ABUSE AMONG LATINOS*

The high rate of drug abuse/dependency among Latinos foretells high rates of negative health and social consequences. Data from the Drug Abuse Warning Network (DAWN), indicates that from 1998 to 2002 Latino emergency department drug episodes increased 67% (from 47,350 to 79,098) (SAMHSA, 2002). This large increase in Latino emergency department episodes does not simply reflect a 67% increase in emergency department episodes but it also includes the broad increase of the Latino population in the United States.

AIDS surveillance data from the CDC indicate that Latino men are more likely to be exposed to HIV through intravenous drug use than white men, and Latina women are more likely to be exposed to HIV by having sex with an HIV positive sexual partner than white women. Researchers attribute this high risk for HIV infection among Latinos and African-Americans to factors such as poverty, low educational attainment, poor access to health care, and high level of intravenous drug use (CDC, 2002). In 2000, Hispanics represented 13% of the U.S. population (including residents of Puerto Rico), but accounted for 19% of the total number of new U.S. AIDS cases reported that year. The percentage of AIDS cases among women was 7% in 1985 and increased to 23% by 1999, and most of this increase has been among Latina women (CDC, 2002). HIV positive Latino men report injection drug use much more frequently than white men do. Latino men with AIDS account for 18% of all male AIDS cases reported in 2002, with 35% reporting injecting drugs, as opposed to white men who account for 47% of all cumulative AIDS cases, with 9% of reporting injection drug use (CDC, 2002). Hispanic women account for 20% of all female AIDS cases and 61% of the female Hispanic AIDS cases can be tied to injection drug use (CDC, 2002).

## *THE ETIOLOGY OF SUBSTANCE ABUSE AMONG LATINOS*

The growing problem of substance abuse among the Latino population over the past fifteen years has resulted in a growing interest in understanding the underlying factors responsible for this increase. These research efforts have resulted in significant advances in understanding the etiology of substance abuse among Latinos (McCuller, Sussman, Dent, & Teran, 2001). Generally, these research advances follow a conceptual framework that views the development of substance abuse behaviors as a process that begins in early adolescence and continues into adulthood (Guo, Hawkins, Hill, & Abbott, 2001). Substance abuse behaviors are viewed as developing by stages initiating with drug experimentation, progressing to drug abuse, followed by addiction, treatment, and relapse (Report by the Commission on Abuse, 1997). Research has also focused on factors influencing or preventing the use or abuse of drugs. Specifically, among Latinos, researchers concentrate primarily on understanding the risk and protective factors associated with the onset of substance abuse among Latino adolescents, and to a lesser extent the development of drug abuse problems among adult Latinos (De La Rosa & White, 2001). Primarily, this research focuses on understanding the role of familial, peer, cultural, and community factors in substance use and abuse among Latino adolescents. Following is a review of the most important studies on the etiology of substance abuse among Latinos.

## *INDIVIDUAL AND FAMILY INFLUENCES*

Research on the role of individual behavioral factors on the use of substances by Latino adolescents is sparse. The few studies that exist have found an association between adolescent substance abuse and such factors as low religiosity, positive attitudes toward drug use, beliefs that drugs are not harmful, low attitudes toward academic achievement including school failure, and participation in deviant behaviors (Brook, Whiteman, Balka, & Cohen, 1997). Psychiatric disorders have been found to be associated with the development of drug dependence among both Latino and non-Latino adolescent and adult populations (Kessler et al., 1997 & 2001). Such comorbidity is independent of race/ethnicity. While there is some research about protective factors at the individual level among white, non-Latino populations (Glantz & Hartel, 1999; Goodman, Simonoff, & Stevenson, 1995;

Luthar, Cushing, Merikangas, & Rounsaville, 1998), there are no known studies that examine individual-level protective factors among Latinos.

The role of familial factors is a relatively well-developed aspect of research on the etiology of substance abuse among Latinos. "Familism" is a uniquely defining trait of Latino culture that is believed to be protective against many negative behaviors, including drug use. Consequently, the lack of family has a profound impact on Latino adolescents. Compared to their African-American and white, non-Latino counterparts from single-parent households, Latino youth have a greater likelihood of becoming alcohol or drug users (Krohn, Lizotte, Thornberry, Smith, & McDowell, 1996; Griffin et al., 2000). Moreover, parent involvement may be more important for Latinos than for other populations studied (Smith & Krohn, 1995). Parental participation in conven tional activities with Latino youth decreases the probability of their using drugs (Krohn & Thornberry, 1993). A study of Puerto Rican youth found that a warm and non-conflicted relationship, identification with the parent, and orientation to parents rather than peers was related to levels of drug use (Brook, Whiteman, Balka, Win, & Gursen, 1997).

## *PEER AND COMMUNITY INFLUENCES*

One of the most consistent and strongest findings is that peer use of alcohol and drugs increases the probability of substance use by youth (Kaplow, Curran, & Dodge, 2002; Windle, 2000). While this is an important etiological aspect, one must be careful not to assume causality, because many young people interested in substances seek out peers who use. Substance use has been found to be higher among Mexican-American students whose friends used drugs than among their peers. In addition, Mexican-American students reported significantly more use of substances when offered by friends (Zapata, Katims, & Yin, 1998). Furthermore, peer drug associations and poly-drug use has been reported to be higher for Mexican American females than for non-Latino white females (Chavez, 1996).

While individual, familial, and peer group factors are important, many patterns of behavior within a given culture or community are collective in nature. The group establishes norms for acceptable behavior, and generally, individuals comply with these group norms. It is, therefore, important to recognize the social and cultural nature of most alcohol and drug consumption and the complex array of external forces that operate to influence patterns of consumption (Straussner, 2001). One observable aspect of a community is alcohol and tobacco advertising in neighborhoods. In 1997, researchers conducted a prevalence survey of outdoor ads in Chicago. Computer mapping was used to locate all 4,247 licensed billboards that were within 500- and 1,000-foot radiuses of schools, parks, and play lots in the city. They found that African-American and Latino neighborhoods were disproportionately targeted for outdoor advertising of alcohol and tobacco (Hackbarth et al., 2001). A contextual analysis of the NSDUH data (Finch, 2001), however, led to the conclusion that neighborhood contexts do not fully explain the variation of alcohol and drug use between Latino and non-Latino white individuals. This study also found that alcohol and drug use varies widely by national origin within Latino groups. This variation was much greater than in the non-Latino groups.

## CULTURAL INFLUENCES

The principal finding about Latino drug use is that U.S.-born Latino adolescents, especially those of Cuban origin, report higher rates of experimental drug use, abuse, and dependence than do other immigrants (Vega et al., 2002). Furthermore, Vega et al., found that identification with, and pride in, any culture may be beneficial; weak cultural identification is associated with greater substance use. Other researchers, such as Felix-Ortiz and Newcomb (1995), found that Mexican-American youth, who were immersed in ethnic activities and reported higher levels of ethnic pride, reported lower levels of substance abuse than other youth. Conversely, Latinos who have become highly immersed in dominant culture, particularly females, are at significant risk for substance use (Gil, Wagner, & Vega, 2000). Among Latino adults, a number of studies have documented the positive relationships between level of acculturation and use of alcohol and other substances (Gil et al., 2000; Vega et al., 1998; Zule et al., 2001).

Researchers have explored the role that stress associated with the acculturation process to American society has upon the drug using behavior of Latinos. Both family and personal stress effects related to acculturation have been found to be risk factors for substance use (Vega, Alderete, Kolody, & Aguilar-Gaxiola, 1998). Additional research is needed to document whether the process of acculturation that results in the erosion of strong family-related protective factors as closeness with parents, traditional Latino values such as respeto (respect for parents) and family pride are related to drug using behaviors of Latino adolescents (Gil et al., 2000).

Clarifying how cultures operate to mediate risk of drug use among Latinos is critical, yet theoretically and empirically challenging. For example, "acculturation" is a multidimensional construct (Oetting & Beauvais, 1987), but most measures lack operational specificity, using, for example, language as a proxy for acculturation level (Escobar & Vega, 2000). In addition, the Latino population is composed of regional groups distributed in accord with historical immigration and migration patterns (Escobar & Vega, 2000).

## *ALCOHOL AND DRUG PREVENTION*

Social scientists have made great strides in understanding and operationalizing knowledge about substance abuse prevention. Most well-known substance abuse prevention programs fall into two basic categories: (1) *Information provision models* such as DARE (Lyman et al., 1999) and the Health Belief Models, and (2) *Social Influence Models* including Life Skills Training (Botvin & Kantor, 2000), the Resistance Strategies Training, such as Project SMART (Hansen, Johnson, Flay, Graham, & Sobel, 1988), Project ALERT (Ellickson, Bell, & McGuigan, 1993), and DRS (Marsiglia, Kulis, & Hecht, 2001). While the impact of information provision models has generally been found to be ineffective, social influence models have been identified as best practice prevention programs by NIDA and CSAP. Meta-analyses of resistance skills training programs support their effectiveness (Tobler & Stratton, 1997).

For over a decade, primary prevention scientists have recognized that risk and protective factors influence outcomes. By focusing on risk and protective factors (including social skills) that are believed to be mutable, prevention efforts aim to eliminate, reduce, or mitigate negative outcomes by interrupting the pathogenic process and enhancing resiliency. Research indicates that tailoring an intervention to a target population can increase its effectiveness (Marsiglia et al., 2000). As a result, there has been an emphasis on ethnically and culturally sensitive prevention programs (Botvin et al., 2000; Schinke, Tepavac, & Cole, 2000).

During adolescence, while youth are undergoing a transitional period of identity and value formation, there are complex interactions between development and cultural context (Harkness & Super, 1983). While there are universal aspects of development such as physical growth, socialization, and shift of referents from adults to peers, these variables interact with culture-specific factors. For example, in a community in which cultural practices include preparing for college, an independent, individuated teenager is not only esteemed, but socially privileged. However, in many Latino cultures where family is a central value, teenagers may opt to stay at home to care for younger siblings. While they are respected for this choice within their culture, they may be viewed by the dominant culture as disadvantaged or socially handicapped in terms of educational goals. Thus, culture cannot simply be viewed as an independent variable-it must be viewed as an integral, dynamic aspect of development (Bronfenbrenner, 1995).

Most prevention programs for non-European ethnic groups are targeted at adolescents who are characterized as "high risk." This is often defined in terms of "low socio-economic status." While economic factors often do influence risk status (Wallace & Bachman, 1991), it would be an oversimplification to reduce substance abuse risk to the issue of socio-economic status. Due to the complexity of adolescents' existence, prevention efforts must consider influences from dynamic, varied social arenas, cultural values, concept/language nuances, and individual characteristics.

Historically, many studies approached ethnicity in a "glossed" fashion, denying the heterogeneity within groups and other contextual factors (Felix-Ortiz & Newcomb, 1995; Straussner, 2001; Trimble, 1995). Acculturation has often been ignored or oversimplified in prevention efforts (Gil et al., 2000). Even when the specific distinction is made, the complexity of acculturative nuances is often overlooked. Specifically among adolescents, studies have found strong relationships between acculturation and substance abuse, with U.S.-born Latino adolescents consistently demonstrating greater ATOD involvement compared with immigrant adolescents (Vega et al., 2002). As research continues to define these cultural groups, causal mechanisms are likely to be found that will help to develop more effective prevention programs. In addition, evidence suggests that Latinos who have become highly immersed in the dominant culture, particularly females, are at significant risk for substance use and related problems (Zapata, Katims, & Yin, 1998). This is an area that needs much more research.

One cannot investigate Latino alcohol and drug abuse without noting the issue of HIV/AIDS transmission. Research in drug treatment centers has found Latino/a HIV prevalence significantly higher in the Northeast and Midwestern regions of the U.S. In addition, some high-risk behaviors associated with drug abuse (such as use of shooting galleries) may be more predominant among Puerto Rico-born Hispanics than among other Hispanics. Recent research also notes that among men, low-acculturation Latinos were significantly more at risk for HIV/AIDS than the other groups, but there was no association between ethnicity and safer needle use among women (Zule, Desmond, Medrano, & Hatch, 2001). It is critical that comprehensive prevention programs include HIV/AIDS prevention messages consistent with values and beliefs of the recipients (CDC, 2003).

## *ALCOHOL AND DRUG TREATMENT*

It is crucial that culture-specific interventions occur across the entire continuum of alcohol- and drug-related services (Delgado, 1999). Marin (1993) defines culturally appropriate interventions as meeting the following characteristics: (1) based on the cultural values of the group, (2) reflect the attitudes, expectations, and norms of the group, and (3) reflect behavior preferences and expectations of group members. Latino natural support systems must be utilized whenever feasible (De La Rosa & White, 2001).

In spite of recent attention to culturally sensitive therapy, little research has been done to assess the effectiveness of various treatment modalities with Latino substance abusers. In fact, the literature has a notable absence of research in this area. There is evidence that current mental health services appear to lack sensitivity to culture. More than half of Latinos using mental health services discontinue therapy after one session (Gloria & Peregoy, 1996). Several reasons for premature termination, including ineffective counseling approaches, a lack of bilingual and bicultural therapists (Glick & Moore, 1990), and failed outreach, recruitment, and retention strategies (SAMHSA, 2002), have been noted.

Using interventions created for non-Hispanic whites and translated into Spanish may not be enough to produce behavior change for Latino clients. Treatment is culturally competent when interventions are based on an understanding of Latino cultural values, when they reflect the client's individual cultural attitudes, expectancies, and norms, and when they respect behavioral preferences (Medina, 2001). Clinicians working with Latino clients can enhance the effectiveness of treatment by understanding and working with the sociopolitical background and cultural values.

One approach to culturally sensitive treatment is Brief Strategic Family Therapy developed at the University of Miami in the early 1970s to reduce problematic behaviors including early substance use. The program, which draws on the natural strength of families and communities, has been found efficacious in randomized clinical trials (Santisteban et al., 2003; Szapocznik & Hervis, 2001). While much work is still needed to develop a full array of effective substance treatment options for Latinos/as, there are several general findings regarding substance treatment to consider when designing treatment for adolescents: (1) the greater the time spent in treatment, the greater the percent of successful outcomes (National Institute on Drug Abuse, 1999; Orlando, Chan & Morral, 2003), and (2) once in treatment, the modes of interventions are fairly comparable in effectiveness, with some added success with family-based interventions (Liddle et al., 2001; National Institute on Drug Abuse, 2001).

## *IMPLICATIONS FOR SOCIAL WORK*

Results from research on the extent and nature of alcohol- and drug-using behaviors of Latinos support the value of utilization of a social network system when providing counseling to Latino clients. Since familial factors play such a central role in alcohol- and drug-using behaviors of Latino individuals, interventions for this population should address the important role of familial factors in the provision of such services.

Social workers developing and providing services to Latino clients need to be aware of the cultural differences existing between the various major Latino subgroups, and even within each of these major groups. For example, the provision of substance abuse counseling services that social workers provide to a recently immigrated 40-year-old male Puerto-Rican experiencing alcoholism problems clearly needs to be different from the services provided to a second-generation 17-year-old Dominican Republic adolescent using cocaine. Moreover, substance abuse programs need to account for the various levels of acculturation to American society found among Latinos.

Since Latinos, particularly males between 21-35-years-old, have higher drug dependency problems than white non-Latinos and African-Americans while having lower access to treatment (Gil-Rivas, 1997), issues of accessibility and retention must be addressed. One strategy is to hire and train staff that reflect the Latino subgroups that the treatment program intends to serve.

Finally, for prevention and treatment practitioners, working with Latino communities requires an appreciation of the dynamics of change-diversification of subgroups within geographic areas; evolving values and norms; acculturation and shifts in family structure; religious affiliations and beliefs; and transitions in attitudes toward and use of alcohol, tobacco, and other drugs. An appreciation of change should be combined with an understanding of deeply rooted beliefs and values that lie at the core of the Latino experience.

Latino communities often are under-served by providers and over-targeted by alcohol advertisers (Hackbarth et al., 2001; Schafer & Caetano, 2001). Exposure to alcohol advertising has been associated with alcohol use (Unger, Schuster, & Zogg et al., 2003).

Consequently, political advocacy aimed at increasing funding levels at the community level may help to alleviate this situation. Communities with more resources have the option of increasing services to the Latino population and regulating the alcohol industry from targeting underage groups.

## *RESEARCH RECOMMENDATIONS*

During the past two decades, many strides have been made in understanding the extent of the drug using behaviors of Latinos living in the United States. What is still unclear is the prevalence of drug use within specific Latino subgroups, such as U.S. born and foreign-born Latinos, and among hidden Latino populations, such as illegal immigrants, Latino gang members, and homeless Latinos. Also unclear is whether the drug using trajectories of Latinos belonging to the various Latino subgroups mirror or differ significantly from those of white, non-Latinos or African Americans (Kandel, 1997). Therefore, needed are population based studies that would address these gaps in the research literature. In addition, we need longitudinal studies that can rigorously test the impact of acculturation related stress on substance using behaviors of Latino populations. The studies that have documented the impact of acculturation related stress on the drug using behaviors of Latinos have been conducted in southern Florida, and involved mostly a sample of U.S.-born individuals of Cuban background (Turner & Lloyd, 2003).

Research studies that delineate the role of protective factors in substance using behaviors are required to fully understand the causal mechanisms. In particular, we need to understand whether such factors as problem-solving ability and positive self-esteem serve as protective barriers against the development of drug using behaviors. Additionally, we need etiological studies that examine community risk factors and the impact they have on the drug using behavior of Latino individuals. For example, drug abuse researchers should examine the relationship between the high rate of female-headed households found in certain Latino communities, such as Puerto Rican communities, and drug using behavior. Also needed are studies that explore the pernicious effects of poverty and whether the effects of such poverty may be neutralized by high levels of residential stability and homeownership in low-income Latino communities (Ross, Reynolds, & Geis, 2000).

Research needs to continue exploring various aspects of prevention and intervention with substance abusing Latinos across the lifespan. It is critical that Latino communities be involved in alcohol and drug research (Delgado, 1999). This needs to occur at all levels including ethnographic investigations, focus groups, curriculum designs, culturally responsive interventions, program improvements, community organizing, and political advocacy. There is a particular need for research that examines acculturation (De La Rosa, 2002) with a more nuanced manner considering the concept orthogonally (Cuellar & Arnold, 1995; Oetting & Beauvais, 1991), as opposed to the oversimplified, linear fashion that has historically been utilized.

## *CONCLUSION*

Data on the prevalence of substance abuse among Latinos indicates that this is a serious problem among Latinos. Beginning in early adolescence, Latinos and Native Americans lead the nation in alcohol and illicit drug use. They also have the highest need for alcohol and illicit drug treatment compared to Whites and African-Americans. As the largest minority in the United States with high fertility and high immigration rates that are expected to continue into the future, there is a need for this nation's institutions to develop effective strategies to address the growing problem of substance abuse among Latinos. These strategies should include at the least: (1) the provision of federal funds to further document the etiology of substance abuse among Latinos, (2) the development of "best practice" drug prevention and treatment models targeting Latino populations, and (3) the dissemination of research findings to those providing prevention and treatment services to Latino populations. Failure by our nation's institutions to take a more proactive approach to countering the growing problem of substance abuse in Latino populations will be detrimental to the future well-being of Latinos and non-Latinos alike.

## NOTES

1. The term "substance use" refers to the lifetime, past year, and past month use of alcohol, cigarettes, marijuana, cocaine, heroin, and other illicit drugs.

2. The term "Latino" refers to the ethnicity of persons who were born or have parents born in any one of the Spanish speaking countries located in South and Central America, or the Caribbean islands (i.e., Mexico, Colombia, Cuba, Dominican Republic, Puerto Rico, etc.). Latinos accept group mores and practices of one's culture of origin with a concomitant sense of belonging.

3. The National Survey on Drug Use and Health (NSDUH), conducted by the Substance Abuse and Mental Health Services Administration (SAMHSA), is a trend study that measures the prevalence of drug and alcohol use among the U.S. household populations ages 12 years and older. The NSDUH is designed to provide annual estimates of alcohol and other drug use among the nation's general population (SAMHSA, 2001).

4. The Monitoring the Future study (MTF) is an annualized survey of 8th, 10th, and 12th grade students living in the United States, excluding students living in Puerto Rico. The study is designed to provide estimates of alcohol and other drug use and of related attitudes and beliefs among the nation's secondary school students (Johnston, O'Malley, & Bachman, 2001). The sampling procedure involves three stages: first, geographic regions are selected; second, schools are selected (without replacement)–approximately 135 schools for twelfth graders, 125 for tenth graders, and 160 for eighth graders; third, students–approximately 49,000 (18,000 eighth graders, 15,000 tenth graders, 16,000 twelfth graders)–are selected from within each school.

## REFERENCES

A report by the commission on substance abuse among America's adolescents (1997). New York: Columbia University.

Anthony, J. C., Warner, L. A., & Kessler, R. C. (1994). Comparative epidemiology of dependence on tobacco, alcohol, controlled substances, and inhalants: Basic findings from the national comorbidity survey. *Experimental and Clinical Psychopharmacology*, 2(3), 244-268.

Beauvais, F., & Oetting, E. R. (2002). Variances in the etiology of drug use among ethnic groups of adolescents. *Public Health Report*, 117(1), S8-S14.

Botvin, G. J., & Kantor, L. W. (2000). Preventing alcohol and tobacco use through life skills training–Theory, methods, and empirical findings. *Alcohol Research & Health*, 24(4), 250-257.

Bronfenbrenner, U. (1995). Developmental ecology through space and time: A future perspective. In *Examining Lives in Context: Perspectives on the Ecology of Human Development.* (Eds.) P. Moen, G. H. Elder, & K. Luscher. Washington, DC: American Psychological Association.

Brook, J. S., Whiteman, M., Balka, E. B., & Cohen, P. (1997). Drug use and delinquency: Shared and unshared risk factors in African American and Puerto Rican adolescents. *Journal of Genetic Psychology*, 158(1), 25-39.

Brook, J. S., Whiteman, M., Balka, E. B., Win, P. T., & Gursen, M. D. (1997). African-American and Puerto Rican drug use: A longitudinal study. *Journal of the American Academy of Child and Adolescent Psychiatry*, 36, 1260-1268.

CDC. (2002). The state of Latinos in HIV prevention community planning: The HIV/AIDS epidemic in the Latino community (electronic data). Atlanta, GA: Center for Disease Control and Prevention.

Chavez, E. L. (1996). Mexican American dropouts and drug use (No. Grant Number DA04777). Rockville, MD: NIDA.

Cuellar, I., & Arnold, B. (1995). Acculturation rating scale for Mexican Americans–II: A revision of the original ARMSA scale. *Hispanic Journal of Behavioral Sciences*, 17, 275-305.

Delgado, M. (1999). Involvement of the Hispanic community in ATOD research. In Mario R. De La Rosa, Bernard Segal, & Richard Lopez (Eds.), *Conducting drug abuse research with minority populations: Advances and issues.* The Haworth Press, Inc., pp. 93-105.

De La Rosa, M., & White, M. (2001). The role of social support systems in the drug use behavior of Hispanics revisited. *Journal of Psychoactive Drugs*, 33, 233-241.

Ellickson, P. L., Bell, R. M., & McGuigan, K. (1993). Preventing adolescent drug use: Long-term results of a junior high program. *American Journal of Public Health*, 83, 856-861.

Epstein, J. A., Williams, C., & Botvin, G. J. (2002). How universal are social influences to drink and problem behaviors for alcohol use? A test comparing urban African-American and Caribbean-American adolescents. *Addictive Behaviors*, 27(1), 75-86.

Escobar, J. I., & Vega, W. A. (2000). Mental Health and Immigration "AAA's": Where are we and where do we go from here? *Journal of Nervous and Mental Disease*, 188, 736-740.

Finch, B. K. (2001). Nation of origin, gender, and neighborhood differences in past-year substance use among Hispanics and Non-Hispanic Whites. *Hispanic Journal of Behavioral Sciences*, 23(1), 88-101.

Gil, A. G., Wagner, E. F., & Vega, W. A. (2000). Acculturation, famialism, and alcohol use among Latino adolescent males: Longitudinal relations. *Journal of Community Psychology*, 28, 443-458

Gil-Rivas, V., Anglin, M. D., & Annon, J. J. (1997). Patterns of drug use and criminal activities among Latino arrestees in California: Treatment and policy implications. *Journal of Psychopathology and Behavioral Assessment*, 19(2), 161-174.

Glantz, M., & Hartel, C. (1999). *Drug abuse: Origins & interventions*. Washington D.C.: American Psychological Association.

Glick, R., & Moore, J. E. (1990). *Drugs in Hispanic communities*. New Brunswick, NJ: Rutgers University Press.

Gloria, A. M., & Peregoy, J. J. (1996). Counseling Latino alcohol and other substance users/abusers: Cultural considerations for counselors. *Journal of Substance Abuse Treatment*, 13(2), 119-126.

Goodman, R., Simonoff, E., & Stevenson, J. (1995). The impact of child IQ, parent IQ and sibling IQ on child behavioral deviance scores. *Journal of Child Psychology & Psychiatry*, 36, 409-425.

Griffin, K. W., Botvin, G. J., Scheier, L. M., Diaz, T., & Miller, N. L. (2000). Parenting practices as predictors of substance use, delinquency, and aggression among urban minority youth: Moderation effects on family structure and gender. *Psychology of Addictive Behaviors*, 14(2), 174-184.

Guo, J., Hawkins, J. D., Hill, K. G., & Abbott, R. D. (2001). Childhood and adolescent predictors of alcohol abuse and dependence in young adulthood. *Journal of Studies on Alcohol*, 62(6), 754-762.

Guzman, B. (2001). *The Hispanic Population*. Washington, DC: U.S. Census Bureau.

Hackbarth, D. P., Schnopp-Wyatt, D., Katz, D., Williams, J., Silvestri, B., & Pfleger, M. (2001). Collaborative research and action to control the geographic placement of outdoor advertising of alcohol and tobacco products in Chicago. *Public Health Report*, 116(6), 558-567.

Hansen, W. B., Johnson, C. A., Flay, B. R., Graham, J. W., & Sobel, J. (1988). Affective and social influences approaches to the prevention of multiple substance abuse among seventh grade students: Results from project SMART. *Prevention Medicine*, 17, 135-154.

Harkness, S., & Super, C.M. (1983). The cultural construction of child development: A framework for the socialization of affect. *Ethos*, 11(4), 221-231.

Hughes, T. L., Day, L. E., Marcantonio, R. J., & Torpy, E. (1997). Gender differences in alcohol and other drug use among young adults. *Substance Use & Misuse*, 32(3), 317-342.

Johnston, L. D., O'Malley, P. M., & Bachman, J. G. (2001). *Monitoring the Future: National Survey Results on Drug Use, 1975-2000*. Bethesda, MD: National Institute on Drug Abuse.

Kandel, D., Chen, M., Warner, L. A., Kessler, R. C., & Grant, B. F. (1997). Prevalence and demographic correlates of symptoms of last year dependence on alcohol, nicotine, marijuana, and cocaine in the U.S. population. *Drug and Alcohol Dependence*, 44, 11-29.

Kaplow, J. B., Curran, P. J., & Dodge, K. A. (2002). Child, parent, and peer predictors of early-onset substance use: A multisite longitudinal study. *Journal of Abnormal Child Psychology*, 30(3), 199-216.

Kessler, R. C., Aguilar-Gaxiola, S., Berglund, P. A., Caraveio-Anduaga, J. J., DeWit, D. J., Greenfield, S. F. et al. (2001). Patterns and predictors of treatment seeking after onset of a substance use disorder. *Archives of General Psychiatry*, 58, 1065-1071.

Kessler, R. C., Crum, R. M., Warner, L. A., Nelson, C. B., Schulenberg, J., & Anthony, J. C. (1997). Lifetime co-occurrence of DSM-III-R alcohol abuse and dependence with other psychiatric disorders in the national comorbidity study. *Archives of General Psychiatry*, 54, 313-321.

Krohn, M. D., Lizotte, A. J., Thornberry, T. P., Smith, C., & McDowell, D. (1996). Reciprocal causal relationships among drug use, peers, and beliefs: A five-wave panel model. *Journal of Drug Issues*, 26, 405-428.

Krohn, M. D., & Thornberry, T. P. (1993). Network theory: A model of understanding drug abuse among African-American and Hispanic youth. In M. De La Rosa & J. L. Adrados (Eds.), *Drug Abuse Among Minority Youth: Advances in Research and Methodology* (Vol. 130, pp. 102-128). Rockville, MD: U.S. Gov. Printing Office.

Liddle, H. A. (2001). Multidimensional family therapy for adolescent drug abuse: Results of a randomized clinical trial. *American Journal of Drug & Alcohol Abuse,* 27(4), 651-687.

Luthar, S. S., Cushing, G., Merikangas, K. R., & Rounsaville, B. (1998). Multiple jeopardy: Risk and protective factors among addicted mothers' offspring. *Developmental Psychopathology*, 10(1), 117-136.

Lyman, D. R., Zimmerman, R. S., Novak, S. P., Logan, T. K., Martin, C., Leukefeld, C. et al. (1999). Project DARE: No effects at 10-year follow up. *Journal of Consulting & Clinical Psychology*, 67, 590-593.

Marin, G. (1993). Defining culturally appropriate community interventions: Hispanics as a case study, *Journal of Community Psychology*, 21, 149-61.

Marsiglia, F. F., Kulis, S., & Hecht, M. L. (2001). Ethnic labels and ethnic identity as predictors of drug use and drug exposure among middle school students in the Southwest. *Journal of Research on Adolescence*, 11(1), 21-48.

Medina, C. (2001). Toward an understanding of Puerto Rican ethnicity and substance abuse. In S. L. A. Straussner (Ed.), *Ethnocultural Factors in Substance Abuse Treatment* (pp. 3-28). New York, NY: The Guilford Press.

McCuller, W. J., Sussman, S., Dent, C. W., & Teran, L. (2001). Concurrent prediction of drug use among high-risk youth. *Addictive Behaviors*, 26(1), 137-142.

National Institute on Drug Abuse. (1999). *Principles of drug addiction treatment: A research-based guide*, NIH Publication No. 99-418.

National Institute on Drug Abuse. (2001). Family based treatment programs can reduce adolescent drug abuse. NIDA Notes: Research findings, 17(4). http://www.drugabuse.gov/NIDA_notes/NNVol17N4/Family.html

Oetting, E. R., & Beauvais, F. (1987). Peer cluster theory, socialization characteristics, and adolescent drug use: A path analysis. *Journal of Counseling Psychology*, 34, 205-213.

Oetting, E. R., & Beauvais, F. (1990-91). Orthogonal cultural identification theory: The cultural acculturation status on delinquency for Mexican-American adolescents. *American Journal of Community Psychology*, 27(2), 189-211.

Orlando, M., Chan, K. S., & Morral, A. R. (2003). Retention of court-referred youths in residential treatment programs: Client characteristics and treatment process effects. *American Journal of Drug & Alcohol Abuse*, 29(2), 337-357.

Ross, C. E., Reynolds, J. R., & Geis, K. J. (2000). The contingent meaning of neighborhood stability for residents' psychological well-being. *American Sociological Review*, 65, 581-597.

SAMHSA. (2001). *Summary of Findings from the 2000 National Household Survey on Drug Abuse* (No. DHHS Publication No. SMA 01-3549). Rockville, MD: Substance Abuse and Mental Health Services Administration.

SAMHSA. (2002). *Drug Abuse Warning Network.* Washington DC: Office of Applied Studies.

Santisteban, D. A., Coatsworth, J. D., Perez-Vidal, A., Kurtines, W. M., Schwartz, S. J., LaPerriere, A., and Szapocznik, J. (2003). The efficacy of Brief Strategic Family Therapy in modifying Hispanic adolescent behavior problems and substance use. *Journal of Family Psychology*, 17(1), 121-133.

Schafer, J., & Caetano, R. (2001). Violence and alcohol: Cultural issues and barriers to treatment. In C. Wekerle & A. M. Wall (Eds.), *Violence and Addiction Equation: Theoretical and Clinical Issues in Substance Abuse and Relationship Violence* (pp. 239-253). New York: Brunner-Routledge.

Schinke, S. P., Tepavac, L., & Cole, K. C. (2000). Preventing substance use among native American youth: Three year results. *Addictive Behaviors*, 25, 387-397.

Schmidley, A. D. (2001). *Profile of the Foreign Born Population in the United States: 2000* (no. P23-206). Washington DC: U.S. Census Bureau.

Sloboda, Z. (2002). Changing patterns of "drug abuse" in the United States: Connecting findings from macro- and microepidemiologic studies. *Substance Use & Misuse*, 37, 1229-1251.

Smith, C., & Krohn, M. D. (1995). Delinquency and family life among male adolescents: The role of ethnicity. *Journal of Youth & Adolescence*, 24, 69-93.

Straussner, S. L. A. (2001). Ethnocultural issues in substance abuse treatment: An overview. In S. L. A. Straussner (Ed.), *Ethnocultural Factors in Substance Abuse Treatment* (pp. 3-28). New York, NY: The Guilford Press.

Szapocznik J., & Hervis, O. E. (2001). Brief Strategic Family therapy: A revised manual. In: *National Institute on Drug Abuse Treatment Manual.* Rockville, MD: NIDA.

Therrien, M., & Ramirez, R. R. (2000). *The Hispanic population of the United States.* Washington, DC: U.S. Census Bureau.

Tobler, N. S., & Stratton, H. (1997). Effectiveness of school-based prevention programs: A meta-analysis of the research. *Journal of Primary Prevention*, 18(1), 71-128.

Trimble, J. E. (1995). Toward an understanding of ethnicity and ethnic identity, and their relationship with drug use research. In G. J. Botvin, S. P. Schinke, & M. A. Orlandi (Eds.), *Drug Abuse Prevention with Multiethnic Youth* (pp. 3-27). Thousand Oaks, CA: Sage.

Turner, R. J., & Lloyd, D. A. (2003). Cumulative adversity and drug dependence in young adults: Racial/ethnic contrasts. *Addiction*, 98, 305-315.

Unger, J. B., Schuster, D., Zogg, J., Dent, C. W., & Stacy, A. W. (2003). Alcohol advertising exposure and adolescent alcohol use: A comparison of exposure measures. *Addiction Research and Theory*, 11(3), 177-193.

Valdez, A., Kaplan, C. D., & Cepeda, A. (2000). The process of paradoxical autonomy and survival in the heroin careers of Mexican American women. *Contemporary Drug Problems*, 27, 189-212.

Vega, W. A., Aguilar-Gaxiola, S., Andrade, L., Bijl, R., Borges, G., Caraveio-Anduaga, J. J. et al. (2002). Prevalence and age of onset for drug use in seven international sites: Results from the international consortium of psychiatric epidemiology. *Drug and Alcohol Dependence*, 68, 285-297.

Vega, W. A., Alderete, E., Kolody, B., & Aguilar-Gaxiola, S. (1998). Illicit Drug Use among Mexicans and Mexican-Americans in California: The Effects of Gender and Acculturation. *Addiction*, 93, 1839-1850.

Wallace, J. M., and Bachman, J. G. (1991). Explaining racial/ethnic differences in adolescent drug use: The impact of background and lifestyle. *Social Problems*, 38(3), 333-357.

Wallace, J. M., Bachman, J. G., O'Malley, P. M., Johnston, L. D., Schulenberg, J., & Cooper, S. M. (2002). Tobacco, alcohol, and illicit drug use: Racial and ethnic differences among U.S. high school seniors, 1976-2000. *Public Health Report*, 117, S67-S75.

Warner, L. A., Canino, G., & Colon, H. M. (2001). Prevalence and correlates of substance use disorders among older adolescents in Puerto Rico and the United States: A cross-cultural comparison. *Drug and Alcohol Dependence*, 63, 229-243.

Windle, M. (2000). Parental, sibling, and peer influences on adolescent substance use and alcohol problems. *Applied Developmental Science*, 4(2), 98-110.

Young, V. D., & Harrison, R. (2001). Race/ethnic differences in the sequences of drugs used by women. *Journal of Drug Issues*, 31(2), 293-324.

Zapata, J., Katims, D., & Yin, Z. (1998). A two-year study of patterns and predictors of substance use among Mexican American youth. *Adolescence*, 33, 391-403.

Zule, W. A., Desmond, D. P., Medrano, M. A., & Hatch, J.P. (2001). Acculturation and risky injection practices among Hispanic injectors. *Evaluation and Program Planning*, 24(2), 207-214.

# Substance Abuse Among Puerto Rican and Dominican Gang Members in a Small City Setting

Mario R. De La Rosa
Douglas Rugh
Patria Rojas

**SUMMARY.** Joining a gang increases an adolescent's risk for substance abuse. To better understand the contextual development of drug use behavior, this retrospective ethnographic study describes a sample of 76 young small-city mainland Puerto-Rican and Dominican males who joined gangs when they were younger. Data is presented and discussed on the drug abuse behavior including their drug using progression and the context in which such use occurs. The young average age of onset 11.2 (sd = 2.6) combined with the rapid progression to more dangerous drugs, which generally occurs within six years, demonstrates the

Mario R. De La Rosa, PhD, is Associate Professor, Florida International University, School of Social Work, 11200 Southwest 8th Street, Miami, FL 33199 (E-mail: mario.de_la_rosa@fiu.edu). Douglas Rugh, MSW, is Research Assistant and PhD candidate, Latino Drug Abuse Research Center, College of Health and Urban Affairs, Florida International University. Patria Rojas, MSW, MPH, is Project Director, College of Health and Urban Affairs School of Social Work, Florida International University.

This research was funded by the National Institute of Health, National Institute of Drug Abuse Grant No. DA014260-01A. All opinions expressed are those of the authors and not of the sponsoring agency.

[Haworth co-indexing entry note]: "Substance Abuse Among Puerto Rican and Dominican Gang Members in a Small City Setting." De La Rosa, Mario R., Douglas Rugh, and Patria Rojas. Co-published simultaneously in *Journal of Social Work Practice in the Addictions* (The Haworth Press, Inc.) Vol. 5, No. 1/2, 2005, pp. 21-43; and: *Substance Abusing Latinos: Current Research on Epidemiology, Prevention, and Treatment* (ed: Mario R. De La Rosa, Lori K. Holleran, and Shulamith Lala Ashenberg Straussner) The Haworth Press, Inc., 2005, pp. 21-43. Single or multiple copies of this article are available for a fee from The Haworth Document Delivery Service [1-800-HAWORTH, 9:00 a.m. - 5:00 p.m. (EST). E-mail address: docdelivery@haworthpress.com].

http://www.haworthpress.com/web/JSWPA

Digital Object Identifier: 10.1300/J160v05n01_02 

elevated risk associated with small city gang membership. Differences in the patterns of drug use were also found between the English and Spanish speaking groups. The authors discuss the implications of the study findings on the development of interventions. Recommendations address future research possibilities on drug abuse within Latino gangs.


**KEYWORDS.** AOD abuse, risk assessment, adolescents, demographic characteristics, Latinos, gang, ethnography research

## *INTRODUCTION*

Joining a gang increases an adolescent's risk for substance abuse. In this paper, the term "substance abuse" includes lifetime, past month, or daily use of alcohol, marijuana, cocaine, and other illicit drugs. Adolescents who join gangs are more likely to abuse drugs than those adolescents who do not join gangs (Cox, 1996; Esbensen, Peterson, Freng, & Taylor, 2002). It is possible that gang entry may be a further developmental step for some boys who are already on a trajectory of worsening antisocial behavior (Lahey, Gordon, Loeber, Stouthamer-Loeber, & Farrington, 1999). However, the trajectory does not appear to be linear and it fluctuates according to the gang's contextual influences. For instance, adolescents who joined gangs were more likely to increase their drug abuse during their period of membership and then decrease their use after leaving the gang (Thornberry, Krohn, Lizotte, & Chard-Wierschem, 1993). Despite the above findings, there continues to be a dearth of research on drug abuse trajectories of gang members. Research over the past decade has concentrated on gang activity within large urban centers such as Los Angeles and Chicago. It is unclear if gang membership increases an adolescent's risk for substance abuse in smaller, less urbanized settings. Furthermore, even though research has demonstrated differences between ethnic groups and substance abuse trajectories, few studies have explored Latino substance abuse within a gang context. Lacking, in particular, are studies that describe Latino adolescents living in small urban communities who may be at risk of joining gangs or who have joined gangs. For the purposes of this article, the term Latino refers to persons of Cuban, Mexican, Puerto Rican, Dominican, or South and Central American descent.

The primary objective of this study is to augment the existing research that has documented the drug abusing behaviors of male Latino gang members. This objective will be accomplished by reporting the findings from an ethnographic study (n = 76) of young small-city mainland Puerto-Rican and Dominican males who joined gangs when they were adolescents and were still involved in gangs at the time they were interviewed. Data from this study on the onset of substance abuse, progression to other drugs, and heavy drug abuse, and the social context in which the onset of substance abuse occurs will be presented and discussed. Implications of the findings for the development of interventions to address the problem of drug abuse among Latino gang members and future research studies on the epidemiology of drug abuse among Latino gangs will be provided.

## *REVIEW OF THE LITERATURE*

Investigations into the lifestyle of Latino gang members received considerable attention by social scientists during the past two decades (Adler, Ovando, & Hocevar, 1984; Hunsaker, 1981; Moore, 1978; Moore, Vigil, & Garcia, 1983). Earlier research on Latino gangs concentrated on the reasons Latino gangs form and the role that these gangs played in the lives of their members (De La Rosa & Caris, 1993). This research found that Latino gangs often supplied emotional and financial support and protection to gang members that was lacking in their families (Moore, 1978; Moore et al., 1983; Vigil, 1983). Drug use, drug selling, and drug related violence was not a primary focus of these studies. Instead these studies examined criminal behaviors associated with gangs. In part, this was due to the fact that during the 70s and 80s drug use and dealing by Latino gang members was mostly individual or small-group behavior which was frequently not sanctioned by other members or leaders (Moore, 1978).

With the development of the crack trade in the late 80s and early 90s, data became available that linked Latino gangs living in large urban areas to the drug trade. Since then there has been a growing interest by researchers to document the drug abuse behaviors and drug-related criminal activities of Latino gangs more extensively. Three empirically based studies have documented the drug abuse behaviors of Latino urban gang members.

Waldorf's (1993) landmark study reported on the drug abuse behaviors of 578 gang members living in a large urban area in the West coast of the United States who were between the ages of 13 to 40 years old. This sample included 293 African-Americans, 157 Latinos (mostly Mexican-American and Salvadorians) and 118 Asian-Pacific Islander gang members. Using conventional questions from the National Household Survey on Drug Abuse detailing weekly, monthly, and lifetime drug use, Waldorf found that Latino gang members abuse illicit drugs more frequently than either African-American or Asian-Pacific island gang members. Data from this study indicated that marijuana was the most frequently used drug during the month prior to the interview regardless of ethnicity or race, followed by heroin, powder cocaine, and crack cocaine. The results also documented that more than 50% of the Latino gang members reported that they felt addicted to a drug sometime in their lives, compared to approximately 25% of African-American gang members.

A second study led by Moore and Hagedorn examined the drug abusing behaviors of 86 male (29 Latinos and 57 African-American) and 69 female (51 Latino and 18 African-American) gang members in a large urban metropolitan area in the Midwest (Hagedorn, Torres, & Giglio, 1998). The majority of the sample was of Puerto Rican descent (75%) and the rest was Mexican-American (25%). Results indicate that for both male and female gang members, alcohol was the most frequently used drug, followed by marijuana and cocaine. Ninety-two percent of the Latino male gang members and 88% of the Latino female gang members reported ever using alcohol, 82% of both the male and female Latino gang members reported ever using marijuana, and 69% of the Latino males and 46% of the Latino female gang members reported ever using cocaine. The onset of drug use for both the male and female gang members in the sample was most likely to begin with tobacco use, progress to marijuana, alcohol, and cocaine. For males, the mean age of onset of tobacco use was 13.8, for marijuana 15.7, alcohol 16, and cocaine 17.8. For the females, the onset of drug use was most likely to begin with marijuana, 15.4, followed by both alcohol and tobacco at 15.8, and cocaine use at 17.3 (Hagedorn et al., 1998).

More recently, Valdez and his colleagues studied the drug using behavior of Mexican-American gang members in a large urban center along the U.S. Mexican Border (Mata et al., 2002). Data collected from 117 active gang members between the ages of 14 to 25 years of age indicate that drug abuse is a serious problem among the interviewed gang members. Data on lifetime alcohol use was reported by 99% of the gang members, 91% used marijuana, 29% used acid/pills, and 48% used inhalants. Results included information on past month use. Sixteen percent of the gang members reported past month crack cocaine use, while 44% reported past month use of powder cocaine, and 13% reported past month use of heroin. Data on past month use of drugs also shows that 77% reported using alcohol, 66% using marijuana, and 9% using inhalants (Mata et al., 2002). The mean range of drug onset begins with marijuana at 12.9-years-old and ends with heroin at 16-years-old.

Data from the above cited studies is similar to that reported by researchers that have documented the onset of substance abuse among high risk adolescents not involved in gangs (DeWit, Offord, & Wong, 1997). In this study, the term "high risk adolescent" refers to youth who have adjudicated as juvenile delinquents, come from families where there is a history of drug use or child abuse, experience academic problems or dropout of school. According to DeWit, Offord, and Wong (1997) research on the drug using behaviors of high risk adolescents not involved in gangs indicates that for these youth the onset of alcohol use begins at age 12 compared to approximately age 16 for lower risk adolescents. Similarly, the onset of marijuana and cocaine use among high risk youth not involved in gangs begins at 15 and 19 years of age compared to the average age of initiation at the ages of 18 for marijuana and 20 for cocaine (Wagner & Anthony, 2002). The results from Wagner and Anthony's study (2002) also suggests that the individuals who initiate alcohol use during early adolescence are often introduced to alcohol by a family member or a close relation with the family within the home.

In summary, the findings from research on the drug using behavior of Latino gang members reinforce the findings on the drug using behaviors of high risk adolescents not involved in gangs. The findings of the present study indicate that the drug using career trajectories of high risk adolescents are much different from those of adolescents in the general population.

## *METHODOLOGY*

### *Sampling Plan and Site*

Seventy-six Dominican and Puerto Rican active gang members were selected and recruited to participate in this study during the years 2001-

2002 using an ethnographically driven targeted sampling approach. The term "active gang member" is used in this study to describe an individual who has been actively involved in gang activities at the time of the interview, including: attending gang meetings, conducting missions for the gangs (e.g., selling drugs, involved in gang-related criminal activity), and having been an integral member of a gang (soldier, leader, etc.). The sampling approach requires that before the identification and recruitment of gang members, community researchers immerse themselves in the neighborhood for the purpose of becoming familiar with the people who live there, observing neighborhood activities, assessing neighborhood safety and receptivity to the research, and determining whether gangs are present. Subsequently, the staff ranked each neighborhood as high, medium, or low on the following criteria: availability of gangs' members, safety, and receptivity to the study. Those neighborhoods that ranked highest across the three categories were selected for further observation.

Puerto Rican and Dominican gang members were recruited from neighborhoods in the city of Lawrence, Massachusetts. Lawrence was selected because it met the study selection criteria of a small city with a high concentration of Latinos. Lawrence is located about forty minutes from the Boston metropolitan area. The 2000 census indicates that 60 percent (43,019) of the 72,043 people that live in the city are of Latino descent. This is about ten times the proportion that lives in the rest of the state (Guzman, 2001). Lawrence's Latino population is also extraordinarily young, resulting in one of the highest proportions of population under the age of 18 in Massachusetts. Lawrence is also one of the most economically depressed communities in the state of Massachusetts, with poverty rates consistently higher than the rest of the state (Jaysane, 2002).

Gang members who voluntarily agreed to be interviewed were selected and interviewed at the community field office or on the street [in another safe location]. An open-ended unstructured interview guide was used. It included the following seven major domains: school adjustments, economic life including future aspirations and goals, family life, gang related activities, substance abuse behavior, involvement with police and criminal justice system, and peer relationships. One gang member was interviewed at one time in order to preserve confidentiality and avoid confrontations between members of rival gangs. All the interviews were recorded and appropriate measures were taken to protect the confidentiality of the data collected. The majority of the interviews lasted approximately two hours.

### *Data Transcription and Analysis*

Several steps were taken to transcribe each two-hour taped interview. Three research staff-persons were involved in the process. Since the data were collected in both Spanish and English, one staff member worked only on the transcription of the English interviews, while the other two staff persons were responsible for transcribing the Spanish interviews. Initially, Spanish interviews were supposed to be translated from Spanish into English for purposes of analysis. This strategy was reworked once the research staff had a sense of the extensive amount of time involved in translation and back translation of the interviews (approximately 90-minute tape interview took approximately 40 hours to transcribe and translate). Due to limited project resources and time, it was decided to maintain the data in Spanish.

Atlas.ti version 4.2 was used for the content analysis. The software made it possible to maintain transcripts in their original form while analyzing the content in English. Using Grounded Theory developed by Glaser and Strauss (1967), the staff identified themes within the data with categories of codes that consistently appeared in the transcribed data. A developmentally informed framework was applied by identifying the interviewer's age. Then the behaviors were identified. By identifying the age in association with a behavior, we were able to track behaviors retrospectively through the growth and development of the individual.

Preliminary analysis of the textual data by three independent analysts revealed that substance abuse was a strong theme in the life of the gang members. Further analyses of the Spanish and English transcripts data provided several categories that offered insights into the drug abuse behaviors of the gang members. The major sub-themes were the following:

a. onset and progression of substance abuse behaviors;
b. types of drugs used;
c. with whom and where drugs were used.

These sub-themes and the coded categories serve as the basis for the comparative analysis of the data presented in this article. Three independent researchers categorized each section of the text by interpreting the meaning of the section. For example, if a person used cocaine at the age of 18-years-old with his girlfriend, the coding protocol for the section would be: 18-years-old, cocaine, and girlfriend. The components of each section can then be analyzed individually or in combination.

Once the themes and sub-themes within the text were identified, the codes were exported to SPSS version 12.0. At this point, each code becomes a variable and the lines of the text converted into cases. The database consists of a document number, a line number, and a dichotomous matrix of zeros and ones. Each instance of the code within the text is marked with a one. An absence of a code results in a zero. Analyses of frequencies are presented below with the results reported for the English speaking sample (n = 38), the Spanish speaking sample (n = 38), and the total (n = 76). The two-group presentation highlights the contrasts and similarities between the Spanish speaking and English speaking groups. The Spanish and English groups were selected depending on whether the interview was conducted in mostly English or Spanish. Nonparametric testing is used for comparing the two groups. Additionally in certain instances associations were tested using the chi square (Phi) test, and group differences were tested between the Spanish and English sub-samples using Mann-Whitney U and Wilcoxon signed-ranked tests, with age as the ranking variable (Daniel, 1995).

### *Sample Demographics*

The sample consisted of 76 males who voluntarily consented to participate in the study. Thirty-eight of the interviews were conducted in Spanish or a mix of Spanish and English and 38 in English only. The sample included 31 (40.7%) gang members born in Puerto Rico; 8 (10.5%) born in Dominican Republic; 1 (1.3%) born in Portugal; and 36 (47.3%) born in mainland United States. The gang member born in Portugal identified himself as a Puerto Rican and therefore was included in the study. Additionally, regardless of where they were born the majority (83%) of the sample grew up in the Northeastern part of the United States. The mean age at the time of the interview of the 62 gang members who reported their ages was 26.7 (sd = 6.7). Thirty-two (42%) of the gang members were married or had a significant other, 28 (37%) were single, and 16 (21%) of the responses were unclear regarding the marital status. Forty-one (54%) of the participants reported having children. The average length of education for this sample is 10 years. Twelve of the gang members who did not graduate from high school completed their Graduate Equivalency Diploma (GED) (see Table 1).

Further analysis of the data, as shown in Table 1, indicates that there were differences in the demographic characteristics of the gang members interviewed in Spanish and those interviewed in English. The results revealed that there were significant differences between the groups (Phi = −.340, p = .01) regarding educational attainment levels suggesting that those individuals whose interview was done in Spanish did not remain in school as long as those individuals who were interviewed in English: The mean years of education were approximately 9.8 years for the Spanish interviewees, and approximately 10.5 years for the English interviewees. The study results also indicate the English speaking sample was more likely born in the mainland United States as compared to the Spanish speaking sample (Phi = .328, p = .02). While there were differences regarding marital status between the English and Spanish sub-samples these differences appear not to be significant.

TABLE 1. Characteristics of Lawrence Gang Members

| | **Spanish Interviews (n = 38)** | **English Interviews (n = 38)** | **Total (n = 76)** |
|---|---|---|---|
| Avg. Age (sd) | 26.9 (6.9) | 28 (6.5) | 26.7 (6.7) |
| Marital Status: | | | |
| Married or Sig. Other | 22 (58%) | 10 (26%) | 32 (42%) |
| Single | 16 (42%) | 12 (32%) | 28 (37%) |
| Unclear | 0 | 16 (42%) | 16 (21%) |
| Have children | 22 (58%) | 19 (50%) | 41 (54%) |
| Born in: | | | |
| Puerto Rico | 18 (47%) | 13 (34%) | 31 (41%) |
| Dominican Republic | 7 (18%) | 1 (3%) | 8 (11%) |
| Portugal | – | 1 (3%) | 1 (1%) |
| In the mainland U.S. | 13 (34%) | 23 (61%) | 36 (47%) |
| Avg. Yrs. of Educ. (sd) | 9.8 (1.6) | 10.5 (2.4) | 10 (2) |

## RESULTS

### *Frequency of Substance Abuse*

Six substances (alcohol, tobacco, marijuana, cocaine, heroin, and pills) were examined and the results are presented. Seventy-four percent of all the gang members in the study have used alcohol at least once in their lifetime, 88% used marijuana, 47% used cocaine, 47% used heroin, 41% used tobacco and 18% used pills sometime in their lives. The majority (82%) reported using more than one drug. Further analysis of the data, as shown in Table 2, revealed slight, nonsignificant differences in the lifetime rate for alcohol, tobacco, marijuana, heroin, cocaine, and pills between the gang members in the English and Spanish subsamples.

The analysis of the data also revealed that 62% of all the gang members reported heavy drug use. The term "heavy drug use" refers to ei-

TABLE 2. Lifetime and Heavy Drug Use Among Gang Members

| By Number (%) | | | |
|---|---|---|---|
| **Lifetime Drug Use** | **Spanish Interviews (n = 38)** | **English Interviews (n = 38)** | **Total (n = 76)** |
| Tobacco | 11 (29%) | 20 (53%) | 31 (41%) |
| Alcohol | 26 (68%) | 30 (79%) | 56 (74%) |
| Marijuana | 33 (87%) | 34 (89%) | 67 (88%) |
| Cocaine | 13 (34%) | 23 (61%) | 36 (47%) |
| Heroin | 12 (32%) | 24 (63%) | 36 (47%) |
| Pills | 7 (18%) | 7 (18%) | 14 (18%) |
| Poly drug users | 29 (76%) | 33 (87%) | 62 (82%) |
| **Heavy Drug Use** | **Spanish Interviews (n = 38)** | **English Interviews (n = 38)** | **Total (n = 76)** |
| **Total Heavy Use** | 25 (66%) | 22 (58%) | 47 (62%) |
| Tobacco | 1 (3%) | – | 1 (1%) |
| Alcohol | 5 (13%) | 17 (45%) | 22 (29%) |
| Marijuana | 15 (39%) | 17 (45%) | 32 (42%) |
| Cocaine | 6 (16%) | 9 (24%) | 15 (20%) |
| Heroin | 13 (34%) | 8 (21%) | 21 (28%) |
| Pills | 1 (3%) | 5 (13%) | 6 (8%) |

ther daily use or at least twice per week use. Forty-two percent of all the gang members reported heavy marijuana use; 29% heavy alcohol use; 28% heavy heroin use; 20% heavy cocaine use; and 8% heavy pill use. It appears that the English-speaking sample used more substances in each category except for heroin.

### *Age of Onset of Substance Abuse*

The results indicate that the average age for the first drug ever used for the entire sample was 11.2 (sd = 2.6) years old. The average age for the onset of tobacco use, 12.8 (sd = 3.8), alcohol use for the entire sample was 12.1 (sd = 3.1), for marijuana use, 13.1 (sd = 2.5), for pill use, 15 (sd = 3.3), for cocaine use, 16.1 (sd = 2.1), and for heroin use, 17.7 (sd = 2.7). Data analysis indicated that among the gang members the average years between the first drug use and the beginning of the last drug was 5.6 (sd = 3.6) (see Table 3).

TABLE 3. Mean Age for Onset of Drug Use Among Gang Members by Types of Drugs

| **Mean (sd) Ages** | | | |
|---|---|---|---|
| | **Spanish Interviews (n = 38)** | **English Interviews (n = 38)** | **Total (n = 76)** |
| Tobacco | 14.6 (4.7) | 11.8 (2.7) | 12.8 (3.7) |
| Alcohol | 12.6 (3.3) | 11.6 (2.9) | 12.1 (3.1) |
| Marijuana* | 13.8 (2.6) | 12.5 (2.2) | 13.1 (2.5) |
| Cocaine | 16.7 (2.6) | 15.8 (1.8) | 16.1 (2.1) |
| Heroin* | 18.8 (2.6) | 17.2 (2.7) | 17.7 (2.7) |
| Pills | 14.7 (2.1) | 15.3 (4.3) | 15 (3.3) |
| Avg. age 1st drug used | 12.3 (2.9) | 10.1 (2.2) | 11.2 (2.6) |
| Avg. number of transitions | 2 (1) | 3 (1.1) | 2.4 (1.1) |
| Average years between first age and last age of onset | 5 (3.1) | 6 (3.9) | 5.6 (3.6) |

*Significantly different age of onset, $p < .05$.

Data on the onset of drug use among the English and Spanish speaking subsamples suggests differences between these two samples. As shown in Table 3, the average age for onset for the first drug used for the English speaking sample was 10.1 (2.2) compared to 12.3 (2.9) for the Spanish speaking sample. The study results also indicate that there were differences in the average age of onset for tobacco, alcohol, marijuana, cocaine, heroin, and pills between the English and Spanish subsamples (see Table 3). It appears that the English speaking sample started to use drugs earlier than the Spanish speaking. Testing this observation revealed that the use of two drugs, marijuana (Mann-Whitney $U = 358$, $p = .01$) and heroin (Mann-Whitney $U = 83.5$, $p = .04$), were significantly different ($p = .05$ level).

The study results also suggest that during their drug abusing years the mean number of transitions (different types of drug use) for all the gang members in the study sample was 2.4 (sd = 1.1). In other words, the average number of drugs reported is three. Among the gang members interviewed in Spanish the mean number of drug use transitions was slightly higher than that of the gang members interviewed in English (see Table 3).

The data from the study also indicates that alcohol (48%) was the most often mentioned drug of choice for first drug used, followed by marijuana (34%) and tobacco (18%). What was occurring in the lives of the interviewed gang members at the time they first used drugs is illustrated by several vignettes taken from the textual data of the gang members interviews and presented below. For the purposes of this article, only vignettes from the interviews in English are included due to the fact that some readers of this article may not be fluent in Spanish and therefore may not be able to fully understand the content of vignettes based upon the interviews conducted in Spanish. The "R" in the vignettes represents the "interviewee's response" to the interviewer questions and "I" represents the interviewer's questions.

A twenty-five-year-old talking about his initiation into the use of heroin:

I: When did you first start using heroin?

R: I was like twenty-three.

I: Tell me about that experience. How did you get introduced to heroin?

R: One night I was real high on crack and that was an upper–I used to sell heroin, but I never used it, but I know that it's a downer, that it will get you down. So I decided to do a bag. I started throwing up.

I: Who was there?
R: Me alone.
I: You were sniffing it?
R: Yeah, me alone I started sniffing it.
I: You were saying you threw up.
R: Then I got used to the high. I stopped throwing up, but then I needed more than a bag to get high, after I picked up a habit.
I: So after about a day or two or three, a week, or two weeks?
R: After like a week I picked up a habit and I needed more to get high. Then I started shooting up.

A thirty-one-year-old man who grew up with two alcoholic parents described his first experience with crack use:

R: I was about nineteen and I had one guy show it to me and he said, look man I ain't got no powder, but I got some crack man, you want some of that. This stuff is ten times better than powder. I'm like, you're kidding me.
I: What'd you think when he told you that? What was going through your mind?
R: Once he said ten times better, my whole body started tingling I'm like ten times–I said it's impossible cause I know what I get the feeling from sniffing. He said, nah man. I'll even give you a hit for free man. You got some money. You wanna buy some if you like it. I said yeah. I had about one hundred and twenty-five. When he seen the money he wasn't like, oh yeah. I could see in his face, he was like oh yeah. That's what I'm saying now cause I know better. I took one hit. It was off of like a little ball. I took that one hit and I held that hit, man cause he told me to hold it.

The study results also suggest that there may be differences in the preferred drug of choice for first drug ever used between the Spanish speaking and English-speaking gang members. For the Spanish speaking gang members as shown in Figure 1, both alcohol and marijuana (42%) were equally preferred for the first drug used, followed by cigarettes (17%). For the English-speaking gang members, alcohol (54%) was the preferred drug of choice, followed by marijuana (27%).

FIGURE 1. Drug of Choice at Onset

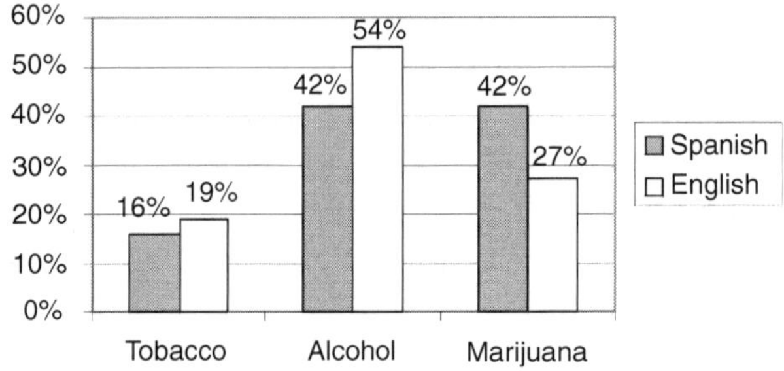


### *Contextual Descriptions*

The analysis of contextual description associated with the onset of substance included information on the gang members' whereabouts at the time they first used any drug and with whom they were at the time of use.

*Who they were with during the onset of drug use?* The study results indicate that forty-eight (63%) of the gang members reported that they were with friends when they first started to use any drug, and 13 (17%) reported that they were with family members. The remaining 13 (17%) gang members reported that they were either with an unrelated person or alone. Among the family members, uncles and stepfathers were among the ones most frequently identified. The important role that friends play in the onset of drug use is highlighted in the vignettes below.

*Friends.* A thirty-one-year-old gang member recounted his first experience smoking cigarettes with his friends as follows:

I: Tell me about the first time you smoked a cigarette?
R: It was cool.
I: How old were you and who was there?
R: Well it was me and my friend Buck and there was whole bunch of us. We were called the Dynamite Kids. At that age I was already like wanting to be. I was a wanna-be. I wanted to be like the other gang, like the older gang member and there was a few of us. There was about eight, nine of us that were the way that I was, not going to

school and just hanging out in the streets. We would just walk around and we'd see cigarettes on the floor or somebody threw cigarette on the floor cause we seen the older guys smoking We'll pick it up and smoke. We'll get a head rush and be like, yeah, this is where it's at.

I: The first time you smoked how was that? How'd you get the cigarette?

R: On the floor, somebody thrown it on the floor. I didn't know who it is, Bird. I seen him throw it on the floor and was like, pick it up and I smoked and I got a head rush and I just went all over telling my friends. Yo, I just smoked a cigarette and then I would just smoke. I would just smoke I would steal my mother's cigarettes and just keep on.

*Family.* Family members also had a significant impact on the onset of drug use behavior among the gang members interviewed as depicted in the excerpts below. A thirty-one-year-old Puerto Rican gang member recounted the first time he drank and the role his family played on his first experience drinking:

I: Do you remember the first time you drank?

R: Oh yeah I was young. I was like four or five-years-old.

I: How'd you get it?

R: My uncles. I would always be up and my moms too, mommy dad and people like that cause I was a hyper person. I was real hyper. I was a bad little kid. Like they would always tell me I was a bad little kid and I was hyper. I was always in and out of things, where I wasn't supposed to be. So to knock me out, give him a sip, give him two, three sips of beers, he'll fall asleep real quick. I believe that's why I became an addict and an alcoholic. I believe that truly.

I: So you tried beer when you were four-years-old and you would have it like when, family occasions?

R: Family occasions, but it was basically everyday. Like I tell you we were living in a house with twelve apartments and out of those twelve apartments, we were renting eight of the apartments.

*Where were the gang members the first time they used drugs?* Thirty-one (41%) of the gang members reported that they were on the street when they first used a drug, which included alleys, parks, woods, and street corners, while 17 (22%) reported that they were in their parents' home, which was most often the mother's home, and 12 (16%) reported that they were in or around school grounds. The remaining 19 (25%) gang members first used in a variety of places, including church, jail, friend's house, and an abandoned building.

*Home.* An excerpt from the gang members interviewed shows just how comfortable some of the gang members felt using drugs in their home during onset. A twenty-four-year-old Puerto Rican gang member discusses where he was when he first drank alcohol:

> I: Were you alone when you tried it?
> R: The first time I was alone. Then like I told a couple of the guys I took a couple sips out of can of beer. Later on in the night I remember I took a wine cooler and I went in the bathroom and I drink it.
> I: At the same party?
> R: At that party yes, later on in the night. I had left the bottle in the bathroom and my older sister went in the bathroom right after I did. She went in there and she'd seen the bottle.The bottle was still cold and it had the frost on it. She knew the bottle was just left there. It wasn't like it was sitting there. The bottle was still cold from being in the icebox. She knew. She was like come here and let me smell your breath. I was like no. She was like I know why and she showed me the bottle. She was like I'll tell, but she never really did.

*School.* A thirty-one-year-old gang member recounting where he was the first time he tried a cigarette:

> I: So where were you? Were you outside the field?
> R: Yeah outside in front of the school. I smoked my first cigarette then. It tasted nasty, gross, but now I'm smoking now, to this day, from that probably. Yeah I didn't smoke weed until like two years later.
> I: Now tell me about cigarettes. How long after did you smoke again, after that first time?
> R: Oh probably, geeze.
> I: Was it an everyday thing or just at football?
> R: No, I think it became like an everyday thing, but at school, not at home.

*Street.* A thirty-two-year-old Puerto Rican gang member recounts the first time he tried alcohol:

I: I wanna hear details. Where were you the first time you tried alcohol?
R: In the street.
I: With whom?
R: With my friends.
I: And they bought it or you?
R: No they bought it. They was older than me. Over there [Puerto Rico] you could buy the beers at the age of 16. I was twelve. So they were older than me. They sell drinks over there. It doesn't matter how old you could be. At the age of sixteen you could buy drink all you want. Here in Massachusetts you buy it at twenty-one. Over there they start buying beers. I started drinking beer, beer, beer. I got home all drunk. I got sick.

*Park.* A thirty-year-old remembers where he started to abuse drugs:

R: I was doing a lot of drinking of hard liquor, like Bacardi was the famous thing to be drinking then, Gin with grapefruit and once in awhile we'll pop some acid pills.
I: Talk to me about the first time you tried that.
R: The first time I tried acid pills, I was in a park. We were hanging out, and it was me, Ricky, Cisco, Pirate, Usano and Polaco and we was gonna initiate this other young kid that he came in the block. We wanted to join us and we was gonna give him in a different way because by this time already I was getting me a kinda tough kid. I really was cocky. I was young. I wasn't scared. I wore my own gun. I had stole it from a car. I learned how to steal from going out with Ricky and stuff.

## *DISCUSSION AND RECOMMENDATIONS*

The results of this study provide one of the first glimpses into the substance abuse behavior of Dominican and Puerto Rican male gang members living in a small city setting. Previous research that has documented the substance abuse behaviors of Latino male gang members (Hagedorn et al., 1998; Mata et al., 2002; Waldorf, 1993) has been conducted in large urban settings. Despite the difference in settings, this study reinforces previous findings that substance use and abuse is a serious problem affecting Latino male gang members regardless of their place of residence. Similar to the previous studies, this study found that the frequency of alcohol, marijuana, as well as cocaine use was very high among gang members (Hagedorn et al., 1998; Mata et al., 2002; Waldorf, 1993).

This study, however, showed some interesting differences in the pattern of drug abuse between gang members in Lawrence and in other cited studies. For instance, the frequency of heroin use was much higher among this study sample than those reported by Mata and colleagues (2002). Additionally, the use of inhalants was almost non-existent among this study's gang members, while the Mata et al. study reported that it was a drug widely used by the gang members in their sample. These results suggest that there is a need to further explore how patterns of substance abuse are affected by the community and geographic area where the gang members reside. There is also a need to further explore whether differences in the patterns of drug abuse are also associated with the ethnic backgrounds of the gang members. While both this study and the Hagedorn et al. (1998) findings were based on data collected from Puerto Rican gang members, the findings reported in Mata et al. and Waldorf (1993) were based on data collected from Mexican, Mexican-American and Salvadorian gang members.

Data on the drug abuse trajectories in this study confirms the findings of previous research on Latino gang members that the onset of drug use and progression to other drugs occurs much earlier among gang members than adolescents in the general U.S. population (Hagedorn et al., 1998; Mata et al., 2002; Wagner & Anthony, 2002). According to Wagner and Anthony (2002), the highest probability for the onset of alcohol and marijuana abuse for the general population is approximately 18 years of age, and the highest probability for the onset of cocaine is two years later. This study suggests that by the age of 16, when most adolescents begin to experiment with illicit drugs, this high-risk cohort has moved into abusing their second or third drug. The earlier onset of drug use among Latino gang members in comparison to the general U.S. population highlights the need for further research to document the underlying factors responsible for such early onset of substance abuse.

The study results also suggest that the drug using career trajectories of the Latino gang members in the sample may differ from most other adolescents. Unlike most adolescents whose onset of drug use typically begins with alcohol or cigarettes before progressing to marijuana and other illicit drugs (Kandel & Faust, 1975), the onset of substance abuse among the gang members in the study begins with alcohol use, followed by marijuana, and tobacco use before progressing to other illicit drugs such as cocaine and heroin. These findings suggest a need for additional epidemiological research to determine whether the drug using career trajectories of Latino gang members follow the same sequence of drug use stages established by the seminal work of Kandel and associates and replicated by other researchers (Elliott, Huizinga, & Menard, 1989; Hops, Tidelsley, Lichtenstein, Ary, & Sherman, 1990). The study results also call for additional research to further document the role of marijuana use in the drug using career trajectories of Latino gang members.

The results generated from this study also raise questions about the role of acculturation in the substance abuse behavior of gang members, since the onset of drug use for first drug used begins at an earlier age for gang members in the English speaking sub-sample in comparison to the Spanish speaking sub-sample (see Table 3). The study also seems to indicate that the age of onset for tobacco, alcohol, marijuana, cocaine, and heroin was younger among the gang members in the English than the Spanish sub-sample. Additionally, the average number of drugs used was higher in English speaking than the Spanish speaking sub-sample. These findings are in line with drug using behaviors among Latino adolescents not involved in gangs (Vega, Gil, & Wagner, 1998). Vega and colleagues found that immigrant Latino male adolescents with low levels of acculturation to U.S. society were more likely to speak Spanish than their acculturated counterparts, and experienced lower levels of both substance abuse initiation and continued drug experimentation than their bicultural or highly acculturated counterparts.

This study also provides strong evidence that friends play a significant role in the onset of substance abuse among the gang members interviewed. Such findings are congruent with the research that has documented the importance of peers in the initiation of substance abuse among adolescents (Duncan, Tildesley, & Duncan, 1995; Windle, 2000).

Finally, this study also demonstrates the capacity that gang members can have in collaborating with researchers in helping elucidate the drug using behaviors of gang members, particular Latino gang members in a small city setting. Future studies should include other Latino ethnic groups and other sites. Replication of this study using other ethnic groups will facilitate knowledge on the progression of drug use among different gang members.

## *IMPLICATIONS FOR SOCIAL WORK*

The results raise several issues about the role of the social work profession in addressing the problem of substance abuse by Puerto Rican and Dominican gang members. The data presented in this article suggests a need for social workers to develop and implement substance abuse prevention, and treatment programs that are multimodal. Multimodal interventions refer to the provisions of services in various settings in the community (e.g., street, home, counseling office, etc.). Prevention efforts must not consider drug abuse and gang membership as facets of the same problem. Interventions may be able to reduce or prevent drug use for male and female gang members while being ineffective in discouraging gang participation, or vice versa. Prevention efforts that incorporate both a gang and a drug component to the intervention will more likely be successful.

Substance abuse prevention programs should target Puerto Rican and Dominican male children at risk of using drugs before they turn age ten. Such programs should include children, family members, and extended family members who are significant to the child. This systemic approach is the starting point for developing effective behavioral responses to prevent their involvement in drug using behaviors. Furthermore, substance abuse prevention programs should target Puerto Rican and Latino families who use drugs but have not yet escalated their drug use to more serious levels.

Social workers should pay particular attention to the use of alcohol, tobacco, and marijuana by family members, and explore ways in which family members can change their drug using behaviors to serve as role models for the children, including referral to appropriate drug treatment services. As previous research has shown, one of the most effective substance abuse prevention strategies among children at risk of abusing drugs is to involve their parents or significant other (Kumpfer, 1999).

Efforts should also be undertaken by social workers to involve Puerto Rican and Dominican children at risk for abusing drugs in appropriate after-school activities. Activities that include children may help to influence the values and attitudes toward drugs and provide a group alternative to joining a gang. Social workers should also seek to develop safe-haven stations within the neighborhood where the high-at-risk Puerto Rican and Dominican children reside and involve parents or a significant other and community gatekeepers in such activities. Services provided under the neighborhood safe-haven stations could range from individual and family counseling to group or individual English tutoring sessions. These services may help to prevent non-English speaking students from becoming isolated.

All of the prevention services must be culturally sensitive and include the provisions of services in the language of the clients. This requires that individuals providing services to Puerto Rican and Dominican children at risk for substance abuse and their families must be fully bilingual. Additionally, the provisions of services should take place in diverse settings (home, school, and counseling office) depending on the need of the family.

Similarly, substance abuse treatment programs need to be culturally sensitive and be ready to address the different levels of acculturation to American society found among Puerto Rican and Dominican gang members and their families. Particularly needed are substance abuse treatment programs that focus on treating poly-drug users as the study results indicate is the case with most of the gang members interviewed. There is also a need to provide treatment to gang members at early stages of drug use in order to prevent the development of more serious patterns of drug use. Such a targeted treatment approach may lead to the prevention of myriad health consequences often associated with long-term drug addiction behaviors (e.g., HIV/AIDS, STD, injury, drug overdose).

The results from this study further augment research on the important role that drug use has in the lives of Latino gang members and suggest that there may be differences in the patterns of drug use among gang members located in different parts of the country that require additional research. The results of this study also call for research that will explore the etiology of drug abuse among Latino gang members, in particular, the role of acculturation.

### *Limitations of the Study*

This study has a number of limitations. The data reported came from a small convenience sample. Therefore, these findings may not be generalizable to other Latino gang members from other parts of the country, or from other ethnic backgrounds. Using interviewers to collect data with a non-structured interviews approach is another limiting factor affecting the veracity of the collected data. While the interviewers were trained to conduct open-ended unstructured interviews, the personal style of the interviewers may have accounted for variations in the data collection. The analysis was not able to control for this bias. While efforts were made to cross-validate the themes and sub-themes that emerged from the content analysis of the transcripts, there was no way to determine whether these themes and sub-themes were artifacts of the coding process, the interviewers, or the analysts.

This study established gang membership by self-report. The self-admitted gang member may be a full member, a 'wannabe,' a former member who still claims to be a member of a gang, or none of these. This study does not provide a measure for the level of gang membership except by the knowledge of the interviewer. Accepting that the gang is a significant factor in drug abuse, it may be important to distinguish the level or intensity of gang membership in developing appropriate treatment and prevention programs.

## REFERENCES

Adler, P., Ovando, C., & Hocevar, D. (1984). Familiar correlates of gang membership: An exploratory study of Mexican-American youth. *Journal of Behavioral Sciences, 6*(1), 65-76.

Cox, R. P. (1996). An exploration of the demographic and social correlates of criminal behavior among adolescent males. *Journal of Adolescent Health, 19*(1), 17-24.

Daniel, W. W. (1995). *Biostatistics: A foundation for analysis in the health sciences* (7th ed.). New York: John Wiley & Sons.

De La Rosa, M., & Caris, L. (1993). The drugs/crime connection among Hispanics: A review of current research. In B. Kail, A. Sachez-Myers & D. Watts (Eds.), *Hispanic and drug abuse* (pp. 81-100): Charles Thomas Printing.

DeWit, D. J., Offord, D. R., & Wong, M. (1997). Patterns of onset and cessation of drug use over the early part of the life course. *Health Education & Behavior, 24*(6), 746-758.

Duncan, T., Tildesley, E., & Duncan, S. C. (1995). The consistency of family and peer influences on the development of substance use in adolescence. *Addiction, 90*, 1647-1660.

Elliott, D. S., Huizinga, D., & Menard, S. (1989). *Multiple problem youth: Delinquency, substance use, and mental health problems.* New York: Springer.

Esbensen, F. A., Peterson, D., Freng, A., & Taylor, T. J. (2002). Initiation of drug use, drug sales, and violent offending among a sample of gang and nongang youth. In C. R. Huff (Ed.), *Gangs in America* (Vol. 3, pp. 37-50). Thousand Oaks, CA: Sage Publications.

Glaser, B. G., & Anselm, L. S. (1967). *The discovery of grounded theory: Strategies for qualitative research.* Chicago, IL: Aldine Publishing Co.

Guzman, B. (May 2001). *Census 2000 Brief: The Hispanic Population.* U.S. Census Bureau.

Hagedorn, J. M., Torres, J., & Giglio, G. (1998). Cocaine, kicks, and strain: Patterns of substance use in Milwaukee gangs. *Contemporary Drug Problems, 25*(1), 113-145.

Hops, H., Tidelsley, E., Lichtenstein, E., Ary, D., & Sherman, L. (1990). Parent-adolescent problem-solving interactions and drug use. *American Journal of Drug and Alcohol Abuse, 16*(239-258).

Hunsaker, A. (1981). The behavioral ecological model of intervention with Chicano gang delinquents. *Hispanic Journal of Behavioral Sciences, 3*(3), 225-239.

Jaysane, A. P. (2002). *The community context of health in Lawrence, Massachusetts.* Lawrence, MA: Merrimack College.

Kandel, D., & Faust, R. (1975). Sequence and stages in patterns of adolescent drug use. *Archives of General Psychiatry, 32*, 923-932.

Kumpfer, K. L. (1999). *Strengthening America's families: Exemplary parenting and family strategies for delinquency prevention.* Retrieved December 30, 2003, from http://www.strengtheningfamilies.org/html/lit_review_1999_toc.html.

Lahey, B. B., Gordon, R. A., Loeber, R., Stouthamer-Loeber, M., & Farrington, D. P. (1999). Boys who join gangs: A prospective study of predictors of first gang entry. *Journal of Abnormal Child Psychology, 27*(4), 261-276.

Mata, A., Valdez, A., Alvarado, J., Capeda, A., Cervantes, R., & Kaplan, C. D. (2002). Drug related violence among Mexican American youth in Laredo, Texas: Preliminary findings. *Free Inquiry in Creative Sociology, 30*(1), 25-39.

Moore, J. W. (1978). *Homeboys: Gangs, drugs, and prison in the barrios of Los Angeles.* Philadelphia: Temple University Press.

Moore, J. W., Vigil, J. D., & Garcia, R. (1983). Residence and territoriality in Chicano gangs. *Social Problems, 31*, 182-194.

Thornberry, T. P., Krohn, M. D., Lizotte, A. J., & Chard-Wierschem, D. (1993). The role of juvenile gangs in facilitating delinquent behavior. *Journal of Research in Crime & Delinquency, 30*, 55-87.

Vega, W. A., Gil, A. G., & Wagner, E. F. (1998). Cultural adjustment and Hispanic adolescents. In W. A. Vega & A. G. Gil (Eds.), *Drug use and ethnicity in early adolescents* (pp. 125-149). New York: Plenum Press.

Vigil, J. D. (1983). Chicano gangs: One response to Mexican urban adaptation in the Los Angeles area. *Urban Anthropology, 12*, 45-75.

Wagner, F. A., & Anthony, J. C. (2002). From first drug use to drug dependence: Developmental periods of risk for dependence upon marijuana, cocaine, and alcohol. *Neuropsychopharmacology, 26*(4), 479-488.

Waldorf, D. (1993). When the Crips invaded San Francisco–Gang migration. *Journal of Gang Research, 1*, 11-16.

Windle, M. (2000). Parental, sibling, and peer influences on adolescent substance use and alcohol problems. *Applied Developmental Science, 4*(2), 98-110.

# Childhood Sexual Abuse and Drug Use Among Low-Income Urban Puerto Rican Women

Mildred Vera
Margarita Alegría
Angela M. Pattatucci-Aragón
Marisol Peña

**SUMMARY.** This study examines the relationship between childhood sexual abuse and adult drug use among low-income urban Puerto Rican women. Interviews were conducted with 718 women, 408 involved in drug use and a comparison group of 310 non drug-users. Results demonstrate a strong association between childhood sexual abuse and adult

---

Mildred Vera, PhD, is Senior Researcher, Center for Evaluation and Sociomedical Research, and Professor, Graduate School of Public Health, Medical Sciences Campus, University of Puerto Rico, P.O. Box 365067, San Juan, PR 00936-5067 (E-mail: mvera@rcm.upr.edu). Margarita Alegría, PhD, is Director, Center for Multicultural Mental Health Research and Visiting Professor of Psychiatry, Harvard Medical School. Angela M. Pattatucci-Aragón, PhD, is Director and Professor, and Marisol Peña, MS, is Researcher, Center for Evaluation and Sociomedical Research, Graduate School of Public Health, Medical Sciences Campus, University of Puerto Rico.

The authors would like to thank María Lebrnó and Abigail González for their support in the preparation of this manuscript.

This research was supported by grant RO1DA09438 from the National Institute on Drug Abuse and grant PO1MH59876 from the National Institute on Mental Health.

[Haworth co-indexing entry note]: "Childhood Sexual Abuse and Drug Use Among Low-Income Urban Puerto Rican Women." Vera, Mildred et al. Co-published simultaneously in *Journal of Social Work Practice in the Addictions* (The Haworth Press, Inc.) Vol. 5, No. 1/2, 2005, pp. 45-68; and: *Substance Abusing Latinos: Current Research on Epidemiology, Prevention, and Treatment* (ed: Mario R. De La Rosa, Lori K. Holleran, and Shulamith Lala Ashenberg Straussner) The Haworth Press, Inc., 2005, pp. 45-68. Single or multiple copies of this article are available for a fee from The Haworth Document Delivery Service [1-800-HAWORTH, 9:00 a.m. - 5:00 p.m. (EST). E-mail address: docdelivery@haworthpress.com].

http://www.haworthpress.com/web/JSWPA

Digital Object Identifier: 10.1300/J160v05n01_03

drug use. The impact of childhood sexual abuse was greater for women reporting greater abuse severity, abuse by a family member, and increased abuse duration. Findings support a direct effects model of childhood sexual abuse on adult drug use. The increased rates of drug use among victims of childhood sexual abuse did not appear to be mediated by other childhood maltreatment or family background factors. Implications for practice and research are discussed. 

**KEYWORDS.** Childhood sexual abuse, women, drug use, Puerto Rico, Latino

## *INTRODUCTION*

Childhood sexual abuse (CSA) is a major health problem that can have a widespread impact over the life of its victims. Beyond the immediate physical and emotional injuries, increased risk for adult substance use has been identified as a long-term health problem associated with CSA (Briere & Elliott, 2003; Chandy, Blum, & Resnick, 1996; Molitor, Ruiz, Klauser, & McFarland, 2000). Numerous investigations with clinical and non-clinical populations have focused on the study of CSA and its effects on adult drug use. Findings with community samples have shown that at least one in five adult women experiences sexual abuse during childhood (Dong, Anda, Dube, Giles, & Felitti, 2003; Finkelhor, 1994, Tjaden & Thoennes, 1998; Finkelhor, Hotaling, Lewis, & Smith, 1990), while estimates among substance abusers have fluctuated from 25% to as many as 75% (Braitstein, Tyndall, Spittal, O'Shaughnessy, Schilder, Johnston, Hogg, & Schechter, 2003; Gil-Rivas, Fiorentine, Anglin, & Taylor, 1997; Grice, Brady, Dunstan, Malcolm, & Kilpatrick, 1995; Medrano, Zule, Hatch, & Desmond, 1999; Paone, Chavkin, Willets, Friedmann, & DesJarlais, 1992; Teets, 1995). Although CSA appears to be more common among women that abuse drugs than for women in the general population, reviews of the research supporting this association point out that it is difficult to compare study findings given the conceptual and methodological differences among studies (Ireland & Widom, 1994; Maman, Campbell, Sweat, & Gielen, 2000). Differences in definitions of CSA, study methods, and sampling procedures all contribute towards the difficulty in understanding the extent and severity of this form of violence against women. This study examines the relationship between childhood sexual abuse and adult drug use among low-income women in Puerto Rico.

A majority of CSA research has focused on non-minority populations. To date, there has been a lack of studies targeting large community samples with solid research methodologies aimed at investigating childhood abuse experiences and drug use among Latino populations. The absence of basic baseline data for Latino populations limits the identification of the magnitude and severity of abuse behaviors in these groups and the capacity to plan appropriate intervention and policy strategies to address their needs. The present study represents an initial step in addressing this issue by examining the prevalence of CSA and its relationship with adult drug use in an urban low-income community sample of Puerto Rican women involved in illicit drug use and a comparison group of women from the same neighborhoods not involved in drug use.

## *REVIEW OF LITERATURE*

One of the major difficulties encountered when attempting to interpret existing data on CSA is the inconsistency in the definition of childhood sexual abuse used in published studies. Childhood sexual abuse definitions have differed on a number of parameters. Depending on the study, the upper age limit used to define victims of CSA can vary from 15 years up to 17 years of age (Ferguson, 1997). Differences are also observed in the type of abusive behavior included in the CSA definition. Behaviors may involve non-contact abuse such as adult exposure; contact abuse that involves touching of genitals or penetration; or some combination of these (Greenberg, 2001). Another parameter that can differ across CSA definitions is the age difference between the perpetrator and the victim, with some definitions setting an age discrepancy (usually the perpetrator must be five years older or more) while others rely on the victim's interpretation of abuse. Although CSA has been documented in many different cultures, the lack of a common definition and other methodological difficulties severely limits the capacity to generalize results eyond specific study populations (Ferguson, 1997; Greenberg, 2001; Mullen et al., 1998).

Variations in sampling frames and measurements also make it difficult to generalize findings across studies. Most of the CSA published studies have sampled from locally defined populations or other discrete groups and there has been no standardized method of data collection or consistent use of comparable, validated outcome measures (Ferguson, 1997). The absence of an appropriate comparison group also limits the value of many studies that examine the relationship between CSA and substance abuse (Ireland & Widom, 1994). Comparison or control groups that enable consideration of relevant variables, such as family background factors, parental substance abuse, and other forms of childhood abuse are essential elements of this research (Bulik, Hettema, Kendler, Myers, Prescott, & Silberg, 2000).

### *Characteristics of the CSA Experience*

A significant body of research sustains the association between CSA and problem behaviors in adulthood; however, it is also known that CSA does not always lead to adverse outcomes. Coffey and colleagues (1996) propose that individual differences in responding to the experience of sexual abuse can be accounted for by the characteristics of the abuse experience itself. Supporting this hypothesis are results from several studies suggesting that the impact of sexual abuse is greater when more invasive sexual acts are involved (Bennett, Hughes, & Luke, 2000; Feinauer, Mitchel, Harper, & Dane, 1996; Ketring & Feinauer, 1999). For example, in a non-clinical, non-student sample of women abused in childhood, Greenwald et al. (1990) observed worse outcomes among victims of incest. Additionally, Freeman and colleagues (2002) report that sexual abuse involving penetration and sexual abuse by a family member are significantly associated with adult drug use. A meta-analysis of studies examining the characteristics of the abuse experience similarly concludes that type of abuse, duration and frequency of the abuse, use of force, and the relationship of the perpetrator with the victim are associated with the number of symptoms reported by victims (Kendall-Tackett, Williams, & Finkelhor, 1993). Overall, these findings highlight the importance of taking into consideration the characteristics of the abuse experience when investigating the relationship between CSA and the development of adverse outcomes as an adult.

### *Childhood Sexual Abuse and Family Environment*

Childhood sexual abuse has been found to occur more frequently in children from socially disadvantaged and disorganized family environments (Fleming, Mullen, & Bammer, 1997; Ferguson, Lynskey, & Horwood, 1996; Mullen et al., 1995; Walsh, MacMillan, & Jamieson, 2003). In a community sample of women, higher rates of sexual abuse were found among those who grew up in unhappy family environments or one-parent households (Finkelhor et al., 1990). Nash and colleagues (1993) produced similar findings and concluded that home environments marked by high levels of disorganization contributed to intensify the effects of CSA, particularly when parents were substance abusers or had criminal backgrounds.

It has been suggested that the linkage between a problematic family background and CSA could be a reflection of lack of sufficient care and supervision, allowing the child to be exposed to the advances of molesters and susceptible to offers of affection (Fleming & Mullen, 1998). Children with disorganized family backgrounds characterized by substance abuse and poor social controls are more likely to come from lower socioeconomic status homes (Buka, Stichick, Birdthistle, & Earls, 2001; Earls, 2001; Earls & Carlson, 2001). Austin (2004) contends that the impact of victimization is particularly harsh for individuals from poor, urban neighborhoods since members of these communities have less access to psychological services and are more exposed to deviant lifestyles, such as prostitution and criminality.

A number of studies have suggested that the relationship between CSA and adult outcomes may not be a simple causal link, highlighting the need to examine potential confounding variables that could influence both the occurrence of abuse and the development of adverse adult outcomes (Singh, Koman, Williams, Catan, & Souply, 1994; Ireland & Widom, 1994; Mullen et al., 1995; Neumann et al., 1996; Mullen & Fleming, 1998). For example, Pedersen and Skrondal (1996) examined this relationship and found that parental substance abuse was associated with both a higher risk of sexual abuse in childhood and with adult substance abuse. They further observed that even after controlling for the effects of parental substance abuse, CSA was significantly associated with adult alcohol abuse. On the other hand, Fleming and colleagues (1998) found that CSA did not have a direct effect on adult alcohol abuse. However, in combination with measures of childhood family environment, being sexually abused did increase the risk of long-term problems. Additional research is needed to further examine the direct and indirect impact of CSA on adult functioning.

### *Childhood Sexual Abuse and Other Forms of Childhood Abuse*

Children who experience one type of abuse have a higher probability of also experiencing other forms of abuse (Dong et al., 2003). For example, Anderson and collaborators (2002) found that women who experienced multiple types of childhood abuse were at increased risk for other negative outcomes compared to women who did not report any experience of childhood abuse. When comparing women who reported either physical or sexual abuse alone to those who reported both physical and sexual abuse, Brown and Anderson (1991) similarly found that those who experienced both forms of abuse were almost twice as likely to report illicit drug use. Mullen et al. (1995) examined the possibility that the associations between CSA and adult difficulties could be accounted for not by CSA itself, but by other forms of abuse (physical or emotional). Findings revealed that even though other forms of abuse accounted for part of the relationship between CSA and problems in adult life, there remained an independent association between CSA and problem behaviors. Overall, the literature presents conflicting findings supporting both the position that childhood sexual abuse has long-term deleterious effects by itself, as well as the position that CSA has a tendency to co-vary with disrupted family backgrounds and other forms of childhood abuse.

The goal of the present study was to investigate the relationship between CSA and adult drug use in an urban low-income community sample of Puerto Rican women involved in illicit drug use and a comparison group of women from the same neighborhoods, but not involved in drug use. The study was designed to address the following questions: (1) what is the prevalence of CSA in a poor, community sample of Puerto Rican drug and non-drug using women; (2) what is the association between CSA and substance abuse and if certain circumstances of CSA might be associated with adult drug use more than others; and (3) what role do other forms of childhood abuse and family environment play in the relationship between CSA and substance abuse?

## *METHODS*

### *Sample Selection and Procedures*

The target population consisted of women, ages 18 to 35, from low-income urban communities in Puerto Rico. Our analysis compares two groups of women: (1) 408 drug users recruited from (a) locations at which illegal drugs or drug paraphernalia are sold or used, known as copping areas, or (b) households within a surrounding 0.2-0.5 mile radius of the copping area, and (2) 310 women who did not meet study criteria for drug use residing within a surrounding 0.2-0.5 mile radius of the copping area.

A two-stage sampling procedure was used to select the copping area sample. Copping areas that sold crack cocaine, powder cocaine, or heroin were identified within inner city communities in Puerto Rico, based on an existing sampling frame developed by Robles, Colón, and Freeman (1993). All 64 copping areas previously identified were visited to assess whether or not they still remained functional and to determine their hours of operation. Copping areas that had closed down, that only operated at night, or did not service female clients were deleted from the list; new copping areas established since the initial identification and that met the selection criteria were added. This process yielded 60 copping areas from which to select study participants. The order in which copping areas were visited by the research team was established through random assignment. The sample was selected from the women who used copping area services between 9 a.m. and 5 p.m. Once the outreach staff arrived at each copping area, they approached all women at the site and explained the purpose of the study. A total of 316 women were approached by the outreach staff, of which 38 were ineligible because of their age and 3 refused to participate. After providing informed consent, 275 female cocaine or heroin users were enrolled in the copping areas for a response rate of 98.8%.

Household sample respondents were selected in a three-stage stratified cluster sampling design with census blocks within a 0.2-0.5 mile radius of inner city drug copping sites as primary sampling units and households as secondary sampling units. Selection was restricted to one woman per household. In a household that had more than one eligible woman, the Kish (1965) random probability selection table was used. A total of 1,653 households was enumerated. From these, 604 eligible women were identified, and 443 interviews were successfully completed, yielding a response rate of 73.3%. Women meeting the criteria for drug use constituted 30% (n = 133) of the household sample.

### *Data Collection*

After obtaining informed consent, data were collected by a private, face-to-face interview conducted at the respondent's house or at a nearby local community center, depending on the respondent's choice. Trained interviewers using a computer assisted interview system that included built-in skip logic and consistency checks conducted the interviews. As a measure of quality control, interviews were tape-recorded. To validate the interview, a random sample of each interviewer's completed interviews was assessed.

### *Measures*

Drug use represented the dependent variable utilized in this study. It was assessed by a positive self-report to use of cocaine (crack or powder) or heroin over the past year or a positive urine or hair test for these drugs. Crack cocaine, powdered cocaine, and heroin were selected as the study drugs due to their popularity among sample women.

The definition of childhood sexual abuse included activities that took place before age 18, with the perpetrator being a family member (regardless of age) or an individual external to the family at least five years older than the respondent. Sexual abuse in this context was operationalized as encompassing any of the following: (1) genital viewing in a sexual context, (2) exposure to pornographic materials, (3) inappropriate touching, grabbing, or kissing, (4) fondling or oral contact of breasts or genitals, (5) digile or penile penetration of the vagina or rectum, and (6) penetration of the vagina or rectum with man-made objects. A series of questions seeking to clarify specific factors of the sexual abuse (i.e., age when abuse began, relationship with perpetrator, and duration) were also asked to examine if certain circumstances of CSA might be related to drug use more so than others. Participants providing affirmative responses to any of the sexual abuse questions were considered to have been sexually abused. A set of dummy variables was created for the measures that assessed the circumstances of the sexual abuse. Type of childhood sexual abuse was organized into four categories: (1) exposure or viewing, (2) inappropriate touching or kissing, (3) fondling or oral contact of breasts or genitals, and (4) penetration. Participants who did not report sexual abuse served as the reference group. When a respondent indicated that she had experienced multiple forms of sexual abuse, she was assigned the code of the act that involved greater physical contact. The dummy variables created for the analysis of the relationship between the victim and perpetrator measured sexual abuse by family members and non-family members. The duration of the sexual abuse was assessed with an open-ended question that allowed responses in units of days, months, or years. Dummy variables created for the analysis measured sexual abuse occurring one day, longer than a day and less than or equal to six months, and in excess of six months. Women with no history of sexual abuse were the reference group for both measures. Those reporting multiple forms of sexual abuse, were assigned the duration and relationship code of the act that involved greater physical contact.

Childhood maltreatment (physical abuse and neglect) and family environment (parental substance use and maternal figure head of household) measures were included in the multivariate analyses to examine their possible mediating effect on the relationship between childhood sexual abuse and drug use. Questions for the measure of physical abuse during childhood were based on the severe violence items included in the Conflict Tactics Scale (CTS PC: Straus, Hamby, Finkelhor, Moore, & Runyan, 1998). Respondents were presented with a series of aggressive actions and asked to report if a mother or father figure had directed the action toward them. The very severe assault actions included hard and repeated beating, burning, or scalding on purpose, threatening with a knife or gun, and grabbing around the neck and choking. Information on other aggressive actions was also collected. These included punching or kicking, hitting with an object, pushing, grabbing or shoving, and slapping. We include the more severe acts of maltreatment in the measure of physical violence. Childhood neglect was assessed with five items from the CTS PC intended to measure failure to engage in behavior that is necessary to meet the developmental needs of a child, such as not providing adequate food, health care, or supervision.

The interview also included questions about socio-demographic characteristics, past year substance use practices, and other health and psychosocial factors. Age, education, annual household income, employment, and marital status were included in all multivariate analyses to control for possible confounding effects.

### *Data Analysis*

Associations between the dependent measure, drug use, and the independent variables were first examined for statistical significance by using chi-square tests. A series of four multiple logistic regression analyses was conducted to assess the independent effects of childhood sexual abuse on adult substance use and examine if some circumstances of CSA might be related to substance abuse more than others. The first set of analyses explored the effect of any childhood sexual abuse on adult functioning. Further logistic regressions attempted to disentangle the impact of (1) each type of abusive act, (2) the relationship between the perpetrator and the respondent, and (3) the length of time over which the abuse occurred. Each set of regression analyses was conducted in two steps. The first step examined the association between each sexual abuse measure and adult drug use adjusting for socio-demographic factors. In the second step, measures of childhood maltreatment and family environment were added to the equations to explore their mediating role in the relationship between CSA and substance abuse. Adjusted odds ratio and corresponding 95% confidence intervals are reported. Results were analyzed using SAS (SAS Institute, Inc., 1999) software.

## *RESULTS*

### *Demographics*

Study participants ranged in age from 18 to 35 years, with a mean age of 27.8 years for participants involved in drug use and 25.4 years for those not involved in drug use. Drug users were older, less educated, more likely to be unemployed or out of the labor force, and never to have married compared to women that did not use drugs (Table 1).

### *Childhood Abuse and Family Conditions*

Although the prevalence of CSA was high for the entire sample, findings revealed significant differences on the childhood abuse measures between women involved in drug use and those that were non-users. Childhood sexual abuse was reported by 35.5% of drug-using participants and 21.3% of women not involved in drug use. A higher proportion of drug using women also reported having experienced physical abuse compared to non-users (39.7% vs. 30.3%). No significant associ-

TABLE 1. Distribution of Demographic and Childhood Factors by Participant's Drug Use

| | Total | | No drug use | Drug use |
|---|---|---|---|---|
| | n | % | % | % |
| Demographic Factors | | | | |
| Age | | | | |
| 18-24 | 269 | 37.5 | 50.3 | 27.7** |
| 25-29 | 181 | 25.2 | 22.3 | 27.5 |
| 30-35 | 268 | 37.3 | 27.4 | 44.9 |
| Education | | | | |
| < High school | 416 | 57.9 | 49.4 | 64.5** |
| ≥ High school | 302 | 42.1 | 50.7 | 35.5 |
| Annual household income | | | | |
| 0-4,999 | 563 | 79.1 | 57.7 | 79.1** |
| ≥ 5,000 | 149 | 20.9 | 42.3 | 20.9 |
| Employment status | | | | |
| Employed | 121 | 16.9 | 24.5 | 11.0** |
| Unemployed | 343 | 47.8 | 44.2 | 50.5 |
| Out of labor force | 254 | 35.4 | 31.3 | 38.5 |
| Marital status | | | | |
| Married | 316 | 44.1 | 54.2 | 36.5** |
| Disrupted marriage | 121 | 16.9 | 13.9 | 19.2 |
| Never married | 279 | 40.0 | 31.9 | 44.3 |
| Childhood factors | | | | |
| Sexual Abuse | | | | |
| No | 507 | 70.6 | 78.7 | 64.5** |
| Yes | 211 | 29.4 | 21.3 | 35.5 |
| Childhood physical abuse | | | | |
| No | 462 | 64.4 | 69.7 | 60.3* |
| Yes | 256 | 35.6 | 30.3 | 39.7 |
| Childhood neglect | | | | |
| No | 457 | 63.7 | 67.4 | 60.8 |
| Yes | 261 | 36.3 | 32.6 | 39.2 |
| Parental substance use | | | | |
| No | 648 | 90.3 | 90.3 | 90.2 |
| Yes | 70 | 9.7 | 9.7 | 9.8 |
| Maternal figure head of household | | | | |
| No | 398 | 55.4 | 58.4 | 53.2 |
| Yes | 320 | 44.6 | 4.0 | 46.8 |

*p < .01 ** p < .001

ations were observed for other childhood measures (childhood neglect, maternal figure head of household, parental substance use). Drug users and non-users were similar in the report of childhood neglect; approximately one third of all study participants indicated that a parent or guardian neglected them. Childhood family conditions were also comparable for drug-using and non drug-using women. Approximately 10% of women in both groups reported substance use by a parent or guardian. Finally, over 40% of drug users and non-users identified a maternal figure as head of household.

### *Circumstances of Childhood Sexual Abuse*

Findings reveal a significant association between specific circumstances of the abuse (type of abuse, relationship of perpetrator to victim, and duration of abuse) and adult drug use (see Table 2).

Women not involved in drug use were less likely to report sexual acts in the more invasive categories compared to drug-using women. Approximately 13% of non-users reported that they were victims of abuse involving manual or oral genital/breast contact (5.8%) or penetration (7.4%), while more than double (27.4%) of the drug using participants reported these experiences (11.5% manual or oral genital/breast contact and 15.9% penetration). The odds of adult drug use were also higher among women who were sexually abused by a family member. Compared to non drug-using women, almost three times more women involved in drug use indicated that they had been sexually abused by a family member (7.9% vs. 20.6%). Similar findings were observed for the measure of CSA duration. Women

TABLE 2. Characteristics of Childhood Sexual Abuse by Participant's Drug Use

| | Total | | No drug use | Drug use |
|---|---|---|---|---|
| | n | % | % | % |
| Type Sexual Abuse | | | | |
| None | 507 | 70.6 | 78.7 | 64.5* |
| Exposure | 43 | 6.0 | 6.1 | 5.9 |
| Inappropriate touching/kissing | 15 | 2.1 | 1.9 | 2.2 |
| Fondling or oral genital/breast contact | 65 | 9.0 | 5.8 | 11.5 |
| Penetration | 88 | 12.3 | 7.4 | 15.9 |
| Relationship of perpetrator | | | | |
| No-abuse | 507 | 72.0 | 80.0 | 65.9* |
| Non-relative | 91 | 12.9 | 12.1 | 13.5 |
| Parent/relative | 106 | 15.1 | 7.9 | 20.6 |
| Duration | | | | |
| No abuse | 507 | 70.6 | 78.7 | 64.5* |
| One day | 111 | 15.5 | 13.6 | 16.9 |
| >1 day < 6 months | 49 | 6.8 | 4.5 | 8.6 |
| > 6 months | 51 | 7.1 | 3.2 | 10.1 |

*$p < .001$

involved in drug use were almost three times more likely to report that the duration of the abuse extended for greater than six months compared to women with no drug use (10.1% vs. 3.2%).

### *Association of CSA and Adult Drug Use*

The results of four sets of regression analyses can be seen in Table 3. Each set of regression analyses was conducted in two steps. The left side of the table shows logistic regression models that examine the independent effects of CSA and specific circumstances of the abuse (type of abusive act, relationship of perpetrator to victim, and duration of abuse) on adult drug use, adjusting for socio-demographic factors. The right side of Table 3 shows results of regression analyses that incorporate

TABLE 3. Logistic Regression: Association of Child Sexual Abuse Related Factors with Adult Drug Use

| | Model 1[a] | | Model 2[a] | |
|---|---|---|---|---|
| | OR | 95% CI | OR | 95% CI |
| A. Any childhood sexual abuse | 2.24 | 1.53-3.37 | 2.17 | 1.45-3.25 |
| Childhood physical abuse | | | 1.29 | .87-1.90 |
| Childhood neglect | | | .88 | .59-1.31 |
| Maternal figure head of household | | | 1.17 | .83-1.65 |
| Parental substance use | | | 1.16 | .66-2.03 |
| B. Type of sexual abuse | | | | |
| Exposure | 1.28 | .63-2.58 | 1.24 | .61-2.52 |
| Inappropriate touching/kissing | 1.27 | .40-4.10 | 1.22 | .37-4.02 |
| Manual or oral genital/breast contact | 2.78 | 1.47-5.23 | 2.74 | 1.43-5.22 |
| Penetration | 2.92 | 1.65-5.15 | 2.82 | 1.57-5.06 |
| Childhood physical abuse | | | 1.30 | .88-1.92 |
| Childhood neglect | | | .88 | .59-1.31 |
| Maternal figure head of household | | | 1.19 | .84-1.67 |
| Parental substance use | | | 1.14 | .65-2.01 |
| C. Relationship of perpetrator | | | | |
| Non- relative | 1.32 | .79-2.20 | 1.29 | .77-2.17 |
| Parent/relative | 3.75 | 2.20-6.40 | 3.64 | 2.10-6.31 |
| Childhood physical abuse | | | 1.31 | .89-1.94 |
| Childhood neglect | | | .88 | .59-1.31 |
| Maternal figure head of household | | | 1.16 | .82-1.64 |
| Parental substance use | | | 1.10 | .62-1.94 |
| D. Duration | | | | |
| One day | 1.63 | 1.02-2.61 | 1.59 | .98-2.59 |
| > 1 day < 6 months | 2.49 | 1.21-5.14 | 2.48 | 1.18-5.20 |
| > 6 months | 4.66 | 2.12-10.23 | 4.47 | 2.00-10.00 |
| Childhood physical abuse | | | 1.25 | .85-1.85 |
| Childhood neglect | | | .90 | .60-1.34 |
| Maternal figure head of household | | | 1.20 | .85-1.69 |
| Parental substance use | | | 1.16 | .66-2.04 |

into the model other childhood factors (physical abuse, neglect, parental substance use, and maternal head of household) that have been identified as potential mediators of the relationship between CSA and drug use.

Findings for the first set of analyses show that the association between any childhood sexual abuse and adult drug use is sustained when controlling for socio-demographic factors. To examine if other childhood factors could be responsible for the observed CSA-adult drug use association, childhood variables related to violence (childhood physical abuse and childhood neglect) and family conditions (female head of household and parental use of drugs) were added to the model. None of these factors explained the childhood sexual abuse-adult drug use association. After controlling for confounding and mediating variables, a direct relationship was sustained. Women who reported being sexually abused as a child were two times (OR, 2.17; 95% CI, 1.45-3.25) more likely to be involved in drug use than women who reported no history of abuse.

It has been suggested that individual differences in responding to the experience of sexual abuse can be accounted for by the characteristics of the abuse experience itself. The second set of logistic regression analyses examined the association between type of childhood sexual abuse and adult drug use. Initial study findings were sustained after controlling for socio-demographic factors. No significant association with drug use was observed among women reporting abusive acts that involved exposure or inappropriate touching or kissing. On the other hand, women reporting abuse by manual or oral genital/breast contact or penetration were almost three times (OR, 2.78; 95% CI, 1.47-5.23 and OR, 2.92; 95% CI, 1.65-5.15) more likely than women reporting no abuse to be involved in drug use. The mediation regression model examined if the association between more invasive childhood sexual abuse acts and adult drug use could be accounted for not by CSA itself, but by other childhood forms of abuse or disrupted family background. Findings supported a strong independent association between more invasive childhood sexual abuse acts and drug use in adult life.

The third set of logistic regression analyses assessed the association between the perpetrator of the sexual abuse and drug use. After controlling for socio-demographic characteristics, women who were abused by a family member were almost four times (OR, 3.75; CI, 2.20-6.40) more likely to use drugs compared to women who were not sexually abused. This association remained significant and did not seem to co-vary when other forms of childhood abuse/neglect and childhood family characteristics were added to the model. On the other hand, the odds of adult drug use were not significantly different for women experiencing CSA by a non-family member in comparison to women who did not report CSA.

Findings for the last set of logistic regression models presented in Table 3 indicate that the length of time over which the sexual abuse occurred is associated with adult drug use. The odds of adult drug use increased according to the duration of the CSA. After adjusting for socio-demographic variables, women who reported that the experience of CSA lasted longer than six months were 4.66 times (95% CI, 2.12-10.23) more likely to use drugs than women who were not sexually abused. Those who reported repeated abuse up to six months were almost two and a half times (95% CI, 1.21-5.14) more likely to use drugs in comparison to women who did not report CSA. When other childhood variables associated with abuse/neglect and family conditions were added to the model this association was sustained. The odds of adult drug use decreased among women who reported having experienced CSA on one occasion. Findings for the mediation regression model show that women who experienced CSA on one occasion had one and a half times the odds of adult drug use as women with no CSA. This association is marginally significant since the confidence intervals narrowly included the null value of 1 (OR, 1.59; 95% CI, .98-2.59).

## *DISCUSSION*

This study examined the relationship between CSA and adult drug use among Puerto Rican women from low-income urban areas. A main goal of this research was to explore the extent to which CSA and adult drug use are related and if certain circumstances of CSA might be associated with adult drug use more than others. This study also investigated if other forms of childhood maltreatment or if certain factors associated with early family environment mediated the relationship between CSA and adult drug use.

Before discussing the findings and implications of this investigation, it is important to address some of its limitations. First, our data are cross-sectional, which allowed us to test relationships between childhood sexual abuse and adult drug use, but not causal pathways. In the case of the childhood measures examined in this study, it seems clear that CSA experiences would have preceded adult substance use. However, these data do not allow us to determine if other factors not measured in the current research might be associated with both childhood sexual abuse and adult drug use. Thus, a prospective study with longitudinal data is needed to further examine our study findings in terms of causal pathways. However, this research may be difficult to carry out because most abused children are not identified. Second, reports of sexual victimization were collected with retrospective self-report that could not be corroborated. There is the possibility that these data might be subject to error from memory fading and reconstruction (Loftus & Ketcham, 1994). Nevertheless, while these factors are important at the individual level, it seems unlikely that they would have had the broad influence, across our cross-sectional sample, necessary to affect significance levels. Supporting this, Hardt and Rutter (2004) argue that such bias is not sufficiently great to invalidate CSA studies that rely on retrospective self-report. Finally, a problem identified by several authors is the lack of consistent measures of CSA across studies (Ferguson, 1997; Greenberg, 2000; Ireland & Widom, 1994; Maman et al., 2000; Mullen et al., 1998). This limits our ability to compare findings from this study on Puerto Rican women to those obtained with other racial/ethnic groups. The field would significantly advance if standardized definitions and measurement tools for CSA were developed. This would facilitate direct comparisons across different studies and would allow for broader conclusions to be drawn.

Notwithstanding these limitations, the current study has a number of strengths. Study data were collected in a culturally sensitive interview format on Puerto Rican women, an understudied population in the CSA research literature. Additionally, this research focuses on a community sample of women involved in drug use and a comparison group that takes into consideration relevant study variables (i.e., ethnicity, socioeconomic status) as opposed to many other CSA studies that have used clinical or student samples. Study participants were recruited from a random sample of drug copping areas and a random household sample in the same low-income urban neighborhoods. This sampling method enabled us to reduce biases attributed to volunteer samples, which may be more willing to disclose abuse and other sensitive issues.

Most CSA studies have been conducted with non-Latino populations. This study represents an initial research effort directed at examining the relationship of CSA and adult drug use with low-income Puerto Rican women. Overall, this study found that the prevalence of CSA was high for both drug-using and non-drug-using Puerto Rican women, 35.5% and 21.3% respectively. However, similar to findings from studies with non-Latino populations (Medrano et al., 1999), results for the present research suggest that CSA is higher among women involved in drug use. Additionally, the prevalence of CSA among non-drug-using Puerto Rican women was also comparable to the rates reported by women in the U.S. (Finkelhor, Hotaling, Lewis, & Smith, 1990; Finkelhor, 1994).

Results for our study population of Puerto Rican women from low-income urban areas demonstrate a strong association between CSA and adult drug use. This finding is consistent with other studies centered on non-Latino samples. A basic focus of our study was to investigate if particular circumstances of CSA might be associated with drug use more than others. Findings reveal that, after controls, the impact of CSA was greater for women reporting the more severe types of childhood sexual abuse, women abused by a family member, and women reporting that the sexual abuse experience extended over a longer period of time. These results are consistent with findings from the meta-analysis conducted by Kendall-Tackett et al. (1993). This study attempted to account for variations in symptomatology by examining characteristics of the abusive experience in 25 independent studies. The authors concluded that abusive experiences involving a perpetrator close to the victim, increased frequency of sexual contact, longer duration, use of force, and sexual practices that included oral, anal, or vaginal penetration lead to a higher number of symptoms for victims.

Although the reasons for involvement in drug use are complex, the research literature offers a number of explanations to account for the link between CSA and adult drug use (Browning & Laumann, 1997; Finkelhor, 1987; Lidberg & Dystad, 1985; Rosenfeld & Lewis, 1993). Finkelhor's (1987) Traumatogenic Model is particularly applicable to our findings. Based on this model, the impact of CSA and the circumstances of the abusive experience can be accounted for through four dynamics: (1) stigmatization, involving messages of badness, guilt, and shame communicated to the child around the abuse, which then become incorporated into his/her image, (2) betrayal, involving the dynamic through which the child realizes that he/she has been caused harm by someone upon whom he/she is fundamentally dependent, (3) powerlessness, conveying the notion in which the child's will and desires are continually disregarded, and (4) traumatic sexualization, referring to the process by which the child's sexuality is shaped in a developmentally inappropriate and dysfunctional way as a result of the abuse.

Our study results can be interpreted within this framework. First, our finding showing increased risk for drug use among adults that were assaulted by someone loved and trusted as children might be due to the sense of betrayal experienced in being harmed by someone charged to protect them. In adulthood, the victim may feel the need to guard from any relationship that could lead to further betrayal. Second, study findings showing worse outcomes among women reporting a longer duration of the abusive experience could be reflective of the powerlessness experienced in not being able to escape and having her will and desires continually disregarded. Coupled with the impact of betrayal, these women might tend to organize any adult relationship around this sense of powerlessness in such a way that being disregarded as an adult recapitulates feelings of worthlessness associated with her CSA. Viewed from this perspective, adult drug use may provide a reasonable means of escape in the mind of the victim, something that she was unable to achieve as a child. Third, our data indicating increased risk for drug use among women reporting more severe types of sexual abuse may lend support to Finkelhor's (1987) notion of stigmatization. Abusive acts involving penetration or genital contact might convey an increased sense of guilt and shame, contributing to poor self-esteem. Despite changing social mores, society values virginity in women and often ascribes its loss to a woman's moral failure–a factor that may be even more extreme for Latinos. In this context, loss of virginity to a family member would represent a profoundly stigmatizing event. This would hold true regardless of whether the CSA remains a secret or is eventually brought to light.

Taken together, we could consider drug use to be one of the coping strategies adopted by CSA victims: (1) to help them distance from the guilt and shame resulting from stigmatization, (2) to facilitate social relationships with minimal interpersonal intimacy (e.g., drug use networks) as a guard from any relationship that could lead to further betrayal, and (3) to numb the memories of abuse and to compensate for the lack of personal power (Bear, Griffiths, & Pearson, 2000; Wilsnack, Vogeltanz, Klassen, & Harris, 1997). Thus, drug use could be viewed as a coping mechanism by which CSA victims distance themselves from painful experiences associated with their childhood trauma. However, it is important to bear in mind that evidence sustaining or challenging the explanations proposed to account for the connections between CSA and adult drug use is sparse (Widom, Weiler, & Cottler, 1999). Clearly, the field needs to undertake more research, in particular with low-income Latino populations, to better understand these complex relationships and refine models of treatment for substance abuse with sexually abused clients.

To address the possibility that CSA might operate primarily as an indicator of troubled family backgrounds, we included other childhood family factors to examine their effect as potential mediators of the relationship between CSA and adult drug use. The present findings support a direct effects model of CSA on adult drug use. After controlling for participants' socio-demographic characteristics, compared to childhood family background (parental drug use and female head of household) and maltreatment factors (childhood physical abuse and childhood neglect), the experience of sexual abuse, as well as the factors related to the circumstances of the abuse (type of abuse, relationship of perpetrator to victim, and duration of the abuse) had a strictly direct (non-mediated) influence on adult drug use. Our findings indicate that the increased rates of drug use among participants with a history of CSA did not appear to be the result of other childhood maltreatment or family background factors, highlighting the importance of CSA and the circumstances of the abuse experience. These observations are consistent with other studies that demonstrate that the effect of CSA over drug use is not mediated by other childhood factors (Downs & Harrison, 1998; Kendler et al., 2000).

The high prevalence of CSA among low-income urban Puerto Rican women and its impact on adult drug use in our sample points to the need for improved prevention, early intervention, and treatment services related to drug use among victims of CSA. Professionals providing care to Puerto Rican women could benefit from being made more fully aware of the extent characteristics, and relationship between CSA and adult drug use. This information would be useful in their clinical work, in order to refer clients to appropriate services, and so that they could become advocates for appropriate training, policies, and resources to provide proper care to the population they serve.

Furthermore, the results of this investigation underscore the importance that drug treatment programs, particularly those providing services to Puerto Rican women, include screening for CSA as a routine component of the intake process. All clients with a positive screening for CSA should be offered a comprehensive assessment (Howard, 2000). Service providers might feel hesitant about screening for CSA for fear of re-traumatizing victims or concerns about their ability to provide care to abused women (Frenken & Van Stolk, 1990). However, several studies report that clients consider it appropriate for health professionals to inquire about physical and sexual abuse and believe that they can be helpful, but indicate that health professionals rarely discuss these topics (Friedman, Samet, Roberts, Hudlin, & Hans, 1992; Greenberg, 2000; Lechner, Vogel, Garcia-Shelton, Leichter, & Steibel, 1993). The Consensus Panel on Substance Abuse Treatment for Persons with

Child Abuse and Neglect Issues (CSAT, 2000) indicates that treatment providers responsible for conducting CSA screening and assessments should receive appropriate training and tools to implement these practices in ways that facilitate opportunities for disclosure. To reduce potential barriers to successful screenings and assessments, they specifically recommend that providers "be sensitive to cultural concerns, recognize potential language differences, become aware of gender issues, and be nonjudgemental and sensitive" (p. 9).

Screening practices for CSA can provide information that is highly relevant for early identification and treatment planning. The Consensus Panel (CSAT, 2000) acknowledges that intervening with child abuse issues while providing treatment for substance abuse can contribute to improve treatment outcomes and reduce the risk of relapse. Interventions specifically directed toward treating the effects of the abuse, paying particular attention to trauma recovery, as a crucial component of care should be considered (Freeman et al., 2002; Goodman & Fallot, 1998). Some of the critical areas which the trauma-focused CSA intervention should pay particular attention to are the enhancement of self-esteem, the management of emotional pain, and empowerment of the individual (Jarvis, Copeland, & Walton, 1998). Future research with Puerto Rican women, as well as other Latinas, is essential to test the relevance and effectiveness of trauma-focused CSA interventions to promote better outcomes for victims of CSA.

## REFERENCES

Anderson, P. L., Tiro, J. A., Price, A. W., Bender, M. A., & Kaslow, N. J. (2002). Additive impact of childhood emotional, physical, and sexual abuse on suicide attempts among low-income African American women. *Suicide Life Threatening Behavior, 32*(2), 131-138.

Austin, A. (2004). Does forced sexual contact have criminogenic effects? An empirical test of derailment theory. *Journal of Aggression, Maltreatment, & Trauma.*

Bear, Z., Griffiths, R., & Pearson, B. (2000). Childhood sexual abuse and substance use. *The Centre for Research on Drugs and Health Behaviour*. Executive Summary. Number 67.

Bennett, S. E., Hughes, H. M., & Luke, D. A. (2000). Heterogeneity in patterns of child sexual abuse, family functioning, and long-term adjustment. *Journal of Interpersonal Violence, 15*, 134-157.

Braitstein, P., Li, K., Tyndall, M., Spittal, P., O'Shaughnessy, M. V., Schilder, A. et al. (2003). Sexual violence among a cohort of injection drug users. *Social Science Medicine, 57*(3), 561-569.

Briere, J., & Elliott, D. M. (2003). Prevalence and psychological sequelae of self-reported childhood physical and sexual abuse in a general population sample of men and women. *Child Abuse and Neglect*, *27*(10), 1205-22.

Brown, G. R., & Anderson, B. (1991). Psychiatric morbidity in adult inpatients with childhood histories of sexual and physical abuse. *American Journal of Psychiatry*, *148*(1), 55-61.

Browning, C., & Laumann, E. (1997). Sexual contact between children and adults: A life course perspective. *American Sociological Review*, *62*, 540-560.

Buka, S. L., Stichick, T. L., Birdthistle, I., & Earls, F. J. (2001). Youth exposure to violence: Prevalence, risks, and consequences. *American Journal of Orthopsychiatry*, *71*(3), 298-310.

Center for Substance Abuse Treatment (CSAT). (2000). Treatment improvement protocol series 36 consensus panel. Substance abuse treatment for persons with child abuse and neglect issues. Rockville (MD): U. S. Department of Health and Human Services, Public Health Service, *Substance Abuse and Mental Health Services Administration*. (Treatment improvement protocol [TIP]) series; no. 36.

Chandy, J. M., Blum, R. W., & Resnick, M. D. (1996). Gender-specific outcomes for sexually abused adolescents. *Child Abuse and Neglect*, *20*(12), 1219-1231.

Coffey, P., Leitenberg, H., Henning, K., Turner, T., & Bennett, R. T. (1996). Mediators of the long-term impact of child sexual abuse: Perceived stigma, betrayal, powerlessness, and self-blame. *Child Abuse and Neglect*, *20*(5), 447-455.

Dong, M., Anda, R. F., Dube, S. R., Giles, W. H., & Felitti, V. J. (2003). The relationship of exposure to childhood sexual abuse to other forms of abuse, neglect, and household dysfunction during childhood. *Child Abuse and Neglect*, *27*(6), 625-639.

Downs, W. R., & Harrison, L. (1998). Childhood maltreatment and the risk of substance problems in later life. *Health Social Care Community*, *6*(1), 35-46.

Earls, F. (2001). Community factors supporting child mental health. *Child Adolescent Psychiatric Clinics of North America*, *10*(4), 693-709.

Earls, F., & Carlson, M. (2001). The social ecology of child health and well-being. *Annual Review of Public Health*, *22*, 143-166.

Feinauer, L. L., Mitchel, J., Harper, J. M., & Dane, S. (1996). The impact of hardiness and severity of childhood sexual abuse on adult adjustment. *American Journal of Family Therapy*, *24*, 206-214.

Ferguson, A. G. (1997). How good is the evidence relating to the frequency of childhood sexual abuse and the impact such abuse has on the lives of adult survivors? *Public Health*, *111*(6), 387-391.

Fergusson, D. M., Lynskey, M. T., & Horwood, L. J. (1996). Childhood sexual abuse and psychiatric disorder in young adulthood: I. Prevalence of sexual abuse and factors associated with sexual abuse. *Journal of the American Academy of Child Adolescent Psychiatry*, *35*(10), 1355- 1364.

Finkelhor, D. (1987). The trauma of child sexual abuse: Two models. *Journal of Interpersonal Violence*, *2*, 348-366.

Finkelhor, D. (1994). Current information on the scope and nature of child sexual abuse. *Future Child*, *4*(2), 31-53.

Finkelhor, D., Hotaling, G., Lewis, I. A., & Smith, C. (1990). Sexual abuse in a national survey of adult men and women: Prevalence, characteristics, and risk factors. *Child Abuse and Neglect, 14*(1), 19-28.

Fleming, J., Mullen, P., & Bammer, G. (1997). A study of potential risk factors for sexual abuse in childhood. *Child Abuse and Neglect, 21*(1), 49-58.

Fleming, J., Mullen, P. E., Sibthorpe, B., Attewell, R., & Bammer, G. (1998). The relationship between childhood sexual abuse and alcohol abuse in women–A case-control study. *Addiction, 93*(12), 1787-1798.

Freeman, R. C., Collier, K., & Parillo, K. M. (2002). Early life sexual abuse as a risk factor for crack cocaine use in a sample of community-recruited women at high risk for illicit drug use. *American Journal of Drug and Alcohol Abuse, 28*(1), 109-131.

Frenken, J., & Van Stolk, B. (1990). Incest victims: inadequate help by professionals. *Child Abuse and Neglect, 14*(2), 253-263.

Friedman, L. S., Samet, J. H., Roberts, M. S., Hudlin, M., & Hans, P. (1992). Inquiry about victimization experiences. A survey of patient preferences and physician practices. *Archival Internal Medicine, 152*(6), 1186-1190.

Gil-Rivas, V., Fiorentine, R., Anglin, M. D., & Taylor, E. (1997). Sexual and physical abuse: Do they compromise drug treatment outcomes? *Journal of Substance Abuse Treatment, 14*(4), 351-358.

Goodman, L. A., & Fallot, R. (1998). HIV risk behavior and poor urban women with serious mental disorders: association with childhood physical and sexual abuse. *American Journal of Orthopsychiatry, 68*(1), 73-83.

Greenberg, J. (2000). Sexual victimization of girls: Implications for women's health and for prevention. In: L. Sherr, J. St. Lawrence (Eds.), *Women, Health, and the Mind.* NewYork: John Wiley & Sons.

Greenberg, J. B. (2001). Childhood sexual abuse and sexually transmitted diseases in adults: A review of and implications for STD/HIV programmers. *International Journal of STD/AIDS, 12*(12), 777-783.

Greenwald, E., Leitenberg, H., Cado, S., & Tarran, M. J. (1990). Childhood sexual abuse: Long-term effects on psychological and sexual functioning in a nonclinical and nonstudent sample of adult women. *Child Abuse and Neglect, 14*(4), 503-513.

Grice, D. E., Brady, K. T., Dunstan, L. R., Malcolm, R., & Kilpatrick, D. G. (1995). Sexual and physical abuse history and post traumatic stress disorder in substance dependent individuals. *American Journal of Addiction, 4*, 297-305.

Hardt, J., & Rutter, M. (2004). Validity of adult retrospective reports of adverse childhood experiences: Review of the evidence. *Journal of Child Psychology Psychiatry, 45*(2), 260-273.

Howard, J. (2000). Substance Abuse Treatment for Persons with Child Abuse and Neglect Issues. Treatment Improvement Protocol (TIP) Series 36, *Substance Abuse and Mental Health Services Administration.* US Department of Health and Human Services: Center for Substance Abuse Treatment. DHHS Publication No. (SMA) 00-3357.

Ireland, T., & Widom, C. S. (1994). Childhood victimization and risk for alcohol and drug arrests. *International Journal of Addictions, 29*(2), 235-274.

Jarvis, T. J., Copeland, J., & Walton, L. (1998). Exploring the nature of the relationship between child sexual abuse and substance use among women. *Addiction, 93*(6), 865-875.

Kendall-Tackett, K. A., Williams, L. M., & Finkelhor, D. (1993). Impact of sexual abuse on children: A review and synthesis of recent empirical studies. *Psychological Bulletin, 113*(1), 164-180.

Kendler, K. S., Bulik, C. M., Silberg, J., Hettema, J. M., Myers, J., & Prescott, C. A. (2000). Childhood sexual abuse and adult psychiatric and substance use disorders in women: An epidemiological and cotwin control analysis. *Archival General Psychiatry, 57*(10), 953-959.

Ketring, S. A., & Feinauer, L. L. (1999). Perpetrator-victim relationship: Long-term effects of sexual abuse for men and women. *American Journal of Family Therapy, 27*, 109-120.

Kilpatrick, D. G., Arcierno, R., Saunders, B., Resnick, H., Best, C., & Schnurr, P. (2002). Risk factors for adolescent substance abuse and dependence: Data from a national survey. *Journal of Consulting Clinical Psychology, 68*(1), 19-30.

Kilpatrick, D. G., & Saunders, B. E. (1997). The prevalence and consequences of child victimization. *National Institute of Justice Research Preview*. Washington, DC: US Department of Justice.

Kish, L. (1965). *Survey Sampling*. New York: Wiley & Sons.

Lechner, M. E., Vogel, M. E., Garcia-Shelton, L. M., Leichter, J. L., & Steibel, K. R. (1993). Self-reported medical problems of adult female survivors of childhood sexual abuse. *Journal of Family Practice, 36*(6), 633-638.

Lidberg, F. H., & Dystad, L. J. (1985). Post-traumatic stress disorder in women who experienced childhood incest. *Child Abuse and Neglect, 9*, 329-334.

Loftus, E., & Ketcham, K. (1994). *The myth of repressed memory: False memories and allegations of sexual abuse.* St. Martin's Press, 283.

Maman, S., Campbell, J., Sweat, M. D., & Gielen, A. C. (2000). The intersections of HIV and violence: Directions for future research and interventions. *Social Science Medicine, 50*(4), 459-478.

Medrano, M. A., Zule, W. A., Hatch, J., & Desmond, D. P. (1999). Prevalence of childhood trauma in a community sample of substance-abusing women. *American Journal of Drug and Alcohol Abuse, 25*(3), 449-462.

Molitor, F., Ruiz, J. D., Klauser, J. D., & McFarland, W. (2000). History of forced sex in association with drug use and sexual HIV risk behaviors. *Journal of Interpersonal Violence, 15*, 262-279.

Mullen, P., & Fleming, J. (1998). Long-term effects of child sexual abuse. *National Child Protection Clearinghouse, Issues in Child Abuse Prevention* (9).

Mullen, P. E., Martin, J. L., Anderson, J. C., Romans, S. E., & Herbison, G. P. (1995). The long-term impact of the physical, emotional, and sexual abuse of children: A community study. *Child Abuse and Neglect, 20*(1), 7-21.

Nash, M. R., Hulsey, T. L., Sexton, M. C., Harralson, T. L., & Lambert, W. (1993). Long-term sequelae of childhood sexual abuse: Perceived family environment, psychopathology, and dissociation. *Journal of Consulting Clinical Psychology, 61*(2), 276-283.

Neumann, D. A., Houskamp, B. M., Pollock, V. E., & Briere, J. (1996). The long-term sequelae of childhood sexual abuse in women: A meta-analytic review. *Child Maltreat, 1*, 6-16.

Paone, D., Chavkin, W., Willets, I., Friedmann, P., & Des Jarlais, D. C. (1992). The impact of sexual abuse: Implications for drug treatment. *Journal of Women's Health I*(2), 149-153.

Pedersen, W., & Skrondal, A. (1996). Alcohol and sexual victimization: A longitudinal study of Norwegian girls. *Addiction, 91*(4), 565-581.

Robles, R., Colón, H., & Freeman, D. (1993). Copping areas as sampling and recruitment sites for out-of-treatment crack and injection drug users. *Drugs and Society, 7*, 91-105.

Rosenfeld, S. & Lewis, D. (1993). The hidden effect of childhood sexual abuse on adolescent and young adult HIV prevention: Rethinking AIDS education, program development, and policy. *AIDS and Public Policy Journal, 8*, 181-186.

SAS Institute Inc. (1999). SAS/STAT® User's Guide, Version 8. Cary, NC: SAS Institute Inc. pp. 1643.

Singh, B. K., Koman, J. J. 3rd., Williams, J. S., Catan, V. M., & Souply, K. L. (1994). Sex differences in self-report of physical health by injection drug users. *International Journal of Addictions, 29*(2), 275-83.

Straus, M. A., Hamby, S. L., Finkelhor, D., Moore, D. W., & Runyan, D. (1998). Identification of child maltreatment with the Parent-Child Conflict Tactics Scales: Development and psychometric data for a national sample of American parents. *Child Abuse and Neglect, 22*(4), 249-270.

Teets, J. M. (1995). Childhood sexual trauma of chemically dependent women. *Journal of Psychoactive Drugs, 27*(3), 231-238.

Tjaden, P., & Thoennes, N. (1998). Prevalence, incidence, and consequences of violence against women: Findings from the National Violence Against Women Survey. *Research in Brief*: Washington, DC: US Department of Justice, Office of Justice Programs, NCJ 172837.

Walsh, C., MacMillan, H. L., & Jamieson, E. (2003). The relationship between parental substance abuse and child maltreatment: Findings from the Ontario Health Supplement. *Child Abuse and Neglect, 27*(12), 1409-1425.

Widom, C. S., Weiler, B. L., & Cottler, L. B. (1999). Childhood victimization and drug abuse: A comparison of prospective and retrospective findings. *Journal of Consultation Clinical Psychology, 67*, 867-880.

Wilsnack, S. C., Vogeltanz, N. D., Klassen, A. D., & Harris, T. R. (1997). Childhood sexual abuse and women's substance abuse: National survey findings. *Journal of Studies on Alcohol, 58*(3), 264-271.

# A Comparison of African American and Cuban American Adolescent Juvenile Offenders: Risky Sexual and Drug Use Behaviors

Jessy G. Dévieux
Robert M. Malow
Emma Ergon-Pérez
Deanne Samuels
Patria Rojas
Sarah R. Khushal
Michèle Jean-Gilles

**SUMMARY.** Racial and ethnic disparities exist in HIV seroconversion rates, with African American and Hispanic youth in the 13-19-year-old

---

Jessy G. Dévieux, PhD, Robert M. Malow, PhD, Emma Ergon-Pérez, MA, Deanne Samuels, PhD, Sarah R. Khushal, MS, and Michèle Jean-Gilles, PhD, are affiliated with the AIDS Prevention Program, College of Health and Urban Affairs, Florida International University, 3000 Northeast 151st Street, ACI 260, North Miami, FL 33181. Patria Rojas, MSW, MPH, is affiliated with the College of Health and Urban Affairs, School of Social Work, Florida International University (E-mail: devieuxj@fiu.edu).

This work was funded in part by Grants RO1 DA 11875 from NIDA and RO1 AA11752 from NIAAA.

[Haworth co-indexing entry note]: "A Comparison of African American and Cuban American Adolescent Juvenile Offenders: Risky Sexual and Drug Use Behaviors." Dévieux, Jessy G. et al. Co-published simultaneously in *Journal of Social Work Practice in the Addictions* (The Haworth Press, Inc.) Vol. 5, No. 1/2, 2005, pp. 69-83; and: *Substance Abusing Latinos: Current Research on Epidemiology, Prevention, and Treatment* (ed: Mario R. De La Rosa, Lori K. Holleran, and Shulamith Lala Ashenberg Straussner) The Haworth Press, Inc., 2005, pp. 69-83. Single or multiple copies of this article are available for a fee from The Haworth Document Delivery Service [1-800-HAWORTH, 9:00 a.m. - 5:00 p.m. (EST). E-mail address: docdelivery@haworthpress.com].

http://www.haworthpress.com/web/JSWPA

Digital Object Identifier: 10.1300/J160v05n01_04

age group representing 61% and 21% of new AIDS cases, respectively. The aim of this study was to examine sexual and drug use behaviors among a sample of 138 African American and Cuban American juvenile offenders. Cuban American adolescents showed higher levels of unprotected sex, higher levels of sex while using drugs, and higher levels of drug/alcohol use in the three and six months prior to confinement. These differences may be explained by multiple factors, including differences in acculturation levels among the Cuban American adolescents, differences in health messages targeted at the two groups, and family mores and norms. 

**KEYWORDS.** HIV/AIDS, African American, Cuban American, adolescents, juveniles, incarcerated, sexual behaviors, drug behaviors

## *INTRODUCTION*

In the United States, significant racial and ethnic disparities exist in HIV rates, with African American and Hispanic youth representing a disproportionate number of cases (CDC, 2002d). Although African American youth comprised only 15% of the 13-19-year age group of adolescents in the U.S., they represent 61% of the new AIDS cases reported in 2000 (CDC, 2002c; Miller, Boyer, & Cotton, 2004). Moreover, Hispanics are also disproportionately represented among adolescents diagnosed with AIDS. For example, during the year 2001 they comprised 15% of the adolescents in the 13-19-year age group in the U.S., yet they accounted for 21% of the newly reported AIDS cases (CDC, 2002c).

Because the Latino community includes people from very diverse regions of Latin America and the Caribbean, the development of well-targeted, effective HIV prevention interventions depends on a clear understanding of these underlying differences. For example, among Hispanics born in Mexico, Cuba, and Central and South America, male-to-male sex appears to be the most prevalent form of HIV transmission (CDC, 2002b). Other data show that among Hispanics born in Puerto Rico, 43% of AIDS cases were related to injection drug use, compared to 6% of cases among Hispanics born in Mexico, and 17% among Hispanics born in the U.S. (CDC, 2002d).

Since many sexually active teens have not been tested for HIV, experts agree that the actual number living with HIV infection is estimated to be much higher than that reported (6,587) (CDC, 2002d; National Institute of Allergy and Infectious Diseases, 2002). Adolescents are often unlikely to protect themselves appropriately and tend to engage in sexual experimentation, often with multiple partners (Henry J. Kaiser Family Foundation, 2002). Many students report using alcohol or drugs when they have sex, and surveillance data suggests that the evaluation of factors influencing the initiation of risk behavior must be ongoing and targeted to specific groups of adolescents (CDC, 2002a). Other research suggests that adolescents rarely use condoms or other barriers during oral sex, considering it to be either "safe" or "abstinence" (Remez, 2000). Minority heterosexual youth in Dade County, Florida warrant special attention where, along with Broward and Palm Beach counties, they comprise 48% of the state's total reported AIDS cases (Florida Annual Report/Epidemiologic Profile, 2002).

In addition to the factors which put minority adolescents at higher risk for HIV infection, previous research has shown that adolescents who have been incarcerated as a result of delinquent behaviors are at higher risk of engaging in sexually risky behaviors than adolescents in the general population (DiClemente, Lanier, Horan, & Lodico, 1991; Kelly, Morgan-Kidd, Champion, & Wood, 2003; St. Lawrence, Crosby, & O'Bannon, 1999). In 1997, ethnic/racial minorities comprised up to one-third of the juvenile population nationwide; however, they represented nearly two-thirds of the detained/committed population in juvenile facilities (U.S. Dept of Justice, 1999). Nationally, the custody rates among Blacks and Hispanics were 1,018 and 515 per 100,000 respectively, compared to 204 per 100,000 among Whites (U.S. Dept of Justice, 1999). The socioeconomic factors, the higher prevalence of AIDS in the minority community, and the overrepresentation of minority youth among the detained/committed population necessitate further research to understand and possibly intervene in the growing HIV epidemic in the adolescent minority population.

The purpose of this study was to examine levels of drug and sexually risky behaviors among a sample of African American and Cuban American adolescent offenders and to assess whether differences between these two groups exist. This study was part of a larger NIH-funded HIV risk reduction intervention among an ethnically diverse sample of detained/confined adolescents in south Florida.

The terms "African-American" and "Black" are used interchangeably to include those individuals who self-identify as either. The term "Hispanic" includes those individuals who self-identify as "Latino/a" or "Hispanic" and also reflects the terminology cited in the literature.

## *METHOD*

### *Participants*

The participants in this study were drawn from a pool of the parent study that included 266 male and 111 female inner city, culturally diverse adolescent offenders enrolled in two ongoing NIH-funded HIV prevention projects conducted in a juvenile detention facility and at a court-ordered treatment center. Participants were recruited from the detention facility and treatment center based on consecutive admissions between 1998-2000. Participants were excluded from the study if they (1) suffered from severe cognitive or psychiatric impairments (e.g., psychosis) that would have compromised their ability to complete the assessment, (2) were not between the ages of 13-19, (3) did not have a history of drug use, (4) refused to provide informed assent and/or their parents (or legal guardians) refused to provide written consent for participation, or (5) were not fluent in spoken English. The sample was limited to 81 African American and 57 Cuban American adolescents found eligible to participate in this phase of the research.

### *Assessment Procedures*

Subsequent to informed assent and parental consent, assessment measures were administered orally to facilitate accurate reporting, full completion, and to compensate for any difficulties in reading comprehension. Each interview lasted approximately 90 minutes. Baseline assessments were administered one week after participants' admission and clearance from treatment staff that detoxification was adequately completed. This procedure was followed to minimize the effect of detoxification or withdrawal factors on test performance and to maximize the accuracy of responses.

Efforts were made to motivate participants to respond accurately, thus reducing the likelihood that reports of sexual experiences were either minimized or exaggerated (Jemmott, Jemmott, & Fong, 1992). Interviewers were careful to ensure that respondents understood the meaning of each question, and repeated or elaborated on questions if a respondent showed any confusion. Participants were informed that their responses were confidential and would be used to help improve HIV prevention programs for other adolescents.

All assessment procedures were conducted by experienced interviewers trained to create a process sensitive to gender and cultural issues. To avoid interviewer drift and other contaminating factors, interviewers received ongoing supervision from a clinical psychologist for the duration of the study. Interviewers were trained to adopt a nonjudgemental attitude during interactions in order to establish rapport and build trust.

### *Measures*

Sex risk and drug risk variables were derived using modified versions of sexual risk assessment measures (Gibson & Young, 1994; Otto-Salaj, Heckman, Stevenson, & Kelly, 1998) that were adapted by Malow and Ireland in 1996 (Malow, Dévieux, Jennings, Lucenko, & Kalichman, 2001). Items included retrospective recall of number of sex partners, unprotected sex acts, and condom use during the previous three- and six-month periods (prior to being in a confined setting), as well as unprotected sex acts proximal to marijuana, alcohol, or cocaine use during those previous three months. Items measuring substance use elicited the frequency of alcohol, marijuana, cocaine, and polysubstance use during the three- and six-month periods prior to being in a restricted environment.

Based on focus groups and in-depth interviews, the research team added items to the survey and modified the language to be culturally sensitive, reflecting the local terminology of the target population. In addition, a tabular format was adapted to facilitate administration and a calendar-based methodology, i.e., a Time-Line Follow-Back Procedure (Sobell, Kwan, & Sobell, 1995; Sobell & Sobell, 1980) was utilized to promote accurate recall.

## *RESULTS*

Independent samples t-tests and chi-square analyses were conducted to determine whether there were differences between African American and Cuban American adolescents on demographic variables, substance use and sexual risk behaviors. (Note: some analyses were not conducted due to small cell size.)

### *Demographics and Delinquent Behaviors*

The total sample included 138 adolescents: 81 African American (59%) and 57 Cuban American (41%). The modal subject was a low-income adolescent who abused alcohol, marijuana, and/or noninjection "crack" cocaine and resided in the inner city. The mean age of the sample was 15.58 ($SD$ = 1.75; range = 13-19), and the average level of education was 8.68 years ($SD$ = 1.56). No significant differences in age existed between the groups but there was a difference in level of education with African Americans having more education ($t$ = 2.90, p = .004) (see Table 1). Eighteen percent of the sample was female. Approximately 15% of the sample lived with both biological parents. For 72% of the Cuban American group, Spanish was the primary language spoken at home.

There was a significant difference between the groups in the number of times illegal offenses were committed (based on self-report), with the Cuban Americans reporting more offenses (t = −2.40, p = .019) (see Table 1). There were no significant differences between the groups in the number of suspensions, expulsions, times picked up by the police, or times arrested.

TABLE 1. Demographics and Delinquency Behaviors

| | African Americans | Cuban Americans |
|---|---|---|
| Sample size | 81 | 57 |
| % female | 17% | 19% |
| Age | 15.6 | 15.56 |
| Education | 9.02 | 8.35* |
| % suspended | 93% | 89% |
| % expelled | 27% | 46% |
| % committed illegal offenses | 80% | 82% |
| Average # offenses | 22.44 | 71.68* |
| % picked up police | 94% | 100% |
| % arrested | 79% | 77% |

* $p \leq .05$

### *Sexual Behaviors*

Significantly more Cuban American adolescents engaged in anal sex than African Americans in the six months prior to detention ($\chi^2 = 14.28$, $p < .001$). Analyses revealed that there were no significant differences between the two groups in the total number of sexual partners, total number of sex acts, total number of vaginal or oral (giving and receiving) sex in the three- or six-month periods prior to program intake.

### *Unprotected Sex*

Cuban American adolescents reported proportionally higher levels of total unprotected sex acts in the three and six months preceding their involvement in the program, compared with African Americans ($t = -2.34$, $p = .021$ and $t = -3.14$, $p = .002$, respectively). Cuban American adolescents reported engaging in proportionally higher levels of unprotected vaginal sex acts during the six months prior to program intake compared with African Americans ($t = -2.01$, $p = .048$). They also reported proportionally higher levels of unprotected oral sex as recipients of such acts in the three and six months preceding their involvement in the program ($t = -2.32$, $p = .022$ and $t = -3.61$, $p < .001$, respectively). Moreover, during the three and six months prior to the program intake, Cuban American adolescents reported proportionally higher levels of unprotected oral sex when giving oral sex ($t = -3.09$, $p = .003$ and $t = -3.93$, $p < .001$, respectively) (see Table 2).

There was no significant difference in the proportion of unprotected vaginal sex acts between the two groups in the three months prior to intake.

### *Drug Use*

The analyses determined that there was a significant difference in combined drug/alcohol use, with significantly more Cuban Americans using substances at three months ($\chi^2 = 8.08$, $p = .006$) and at six months ($\chi^2 = 13.30$, $p < .001$) prior to detention. At six months prior to program admission 93% of Cuban Americans had used alcohol/drugs compared with 67% of the African American adolescents. There was a significant difference in the number of times multiple substances were used in the previous six months, with Cuban Americans on average using multiple

TABLE 2. T-Test Comparisons of Sex and Drug Use Behaviors-Significant Results

| Variable | African American (n = 81) Mean (SD) | Cuban American (n = 57) Mean (SD) | *t* | p |
|---|---|---|---|---|
| Proportion Unprotected Vaginal Sex Acts (6 months) | 17.95(32.90) | 30.89(40.17) | −2.01 | .048 |
| Proportion Unprotected Oral Receiving Sex Acts (3 months) | 24.90(42.77) | 43.86(50.06) | −2.32 | .022 |
| Proportion Unprotected Oral Receiving Sex Acts (6 months) | 23.29(41.70) | 52.63(50.37) | −3.61 | .000 |
| Proportion Unprotected Oral Giving Sex Acts (3 months) | 7.41(26.35) | 28.07(45.33) | −3.09 | .003 |
| Proportion Unprotected Oral Giving Sex Acts (6 months) | 8.64(28.27) | 36.84(48.67) | −3.93 | .000 |
| Total Proportion Unprotected Sex Acts (3 months) | 26.37(36.73) | 42.08(41.60) | −2.34 | .021 |
| Total Proportion Unprotected Sex Acts (6 months) | 24.11(35.38) | 44.31(39.61) | −3.14 | .002 |
| Number of Times Used Multiple Substances (6 months) | 7.49(25.11) | 21.09(38.48) | −2.34 | .022 |
| Proportion Unprotected Sex when High on Alcohol (3 months) | 4.66(20.25) | 15.59(35.39) | −2.10 | .039 |
| Proportion Unprotected Sex when High on Polysubstances (3 months) | 1.96(12.38) | 14.78(35.19) | −2.64 | .010 |

drugs more often than African Americans ($t = -2.34$, $p = .022$) (see Table 2).

There were no significant differences in the number of times the two groups of adolescents used specific substances (alcohol, marijuana, or cocaine) in the three and six months prior to their intake. There was also no significant difference in total drug/alcohol use by group or multiple drug use in the previous three months.

### *Sex and Drugs*

Cuban American adolescents reported engaging in proportionally higher levels of unprotected sex acts, compared with African Americans, when high on alcohol ($t = -2.10$, $p = .039$), and higher levels of unprotected sex acts when high on two or more drugs ($t = -2.64$, $p = .010$)

during the three months prior to program intake. There were no significant differences between the two groups in the proportion of unprotected sex when high on cocaine or marijuana in the three months prior to intake (see Table 2).

## *DISCUSSION*

The results show that within this sample of confined, low income, African American and Cuban American adolescents, there were high levels of engagement in risky behaviors that could potentially lead to HIV infection. There were many areas of commonality between the two groups, most notably in their levels of sexual activity and number of partners. These findings differ somewhat from a study conducted among a nationally representative sample of adolescents, which showed that Blacks were more likely to engage in sex and have a higher number of sexual partners than their Hispanic counterparts (Grunbaum et al., 2002). It should be noted, however, that in the national sample, data for Hispanics represented the combination of all Hispanic subgroups, and thus the relative contribution of each subgroup could not be determined.

In those areas for which significant differences were found, there were higher levels of unprotected sex and higher levels of sex while using drugs among Cuban American adolescents. These findings reflect the findings in the national sample which showed that, compared with Whites and Hispanics, Blacks were significantly more likely to have used condoms at last sex and were also less likely to use alcohol and drugs during the last sexual episode (Grunbaum et al., 2002). Cuban American adolescents in this sample reported significantly more illegal offenses than the African American adolescents, and a greater percentage had used drugs/alcohol in the past six months (93% vs. 67%) suggesting perhaps that they represent a more hardened group of delinquents than the African American sample. These findings may in part explain the higher level of engagement in risky behaviors among the Cuban Americans.

Although much research has been devoted to studying Hispanic adolescents' engagement in risky behaviors, data for this very diverse population have often been pooled, thereby obscuring areas of wide divergence among the groups. An important element in these studies has been the issue of acculturation. Research has shown that acculturation, and issues surrounding inter-generational conflict are important factors in the delinquent behavior of Hispanic youth (e.g., Vega, Gil, Warheit, Zimmerman, & Apospori, 1993). Studies have shown, for example, that adolescents who are more acculturated engage earlier and more frequently in risky behaviors than their less acculturated counterparts (e.g., Vega, Gil, & Zimmerman, 1993). Another study revealed that White and U.S. born Hispanic adolescents in south Florida had the highest lifetime and past year prevalence of substance abuse (Khoury, Warheit, & Zimmerman, 1996) compared with other ethnic groups.

Due to the limited number of items assessing acculturation in the current study, further analyses on this topic were not possible; however, acculturation effects may in part explain the higher levels of engagement in risky behaviors by the Cuban American adolescents in this sample. Studies have shown that youth who have immigrated to the U.S. or who were born to immigrant parents feel greater peer pressure to engage in substance abuse and sexual activity (e.g., Blake, Ledsky, Goodenow, & O'Donnell, 2001). Other work suggests that U.S. born Latino adolescents who have acculturated are more likely to exhibit problematic risk behaviors than foreign born and less acculturated Latino adolescents (Ebin, Sneed, Morisky, Rotheram-Borus, Magnusson, & Malotte, 2001) and that more acculturated Latino youth have higher rates of drug use than Latino immigrants (Unger et al., 2000). These empirical results point to the importance of studying the impact of acculturation; further studies are needed to understand its relative contribution to risky behaviors.

The differences between African American and Cuban American adolescents may additionally be due to the differences in targeted efforts and specific messages directed towards each of these subgroups. Given that the level of HIV among African Americans has been rising dramatically, much media attention as well as attention by a host of researchers/clinicians has been focused on African American youth to prevent increased levels of the disease in this population. Although the Cuban American adolescents in this study were all fluent in English, it is possible that they, as a separate and distinct cultural group, have not been targeted, to the extent seen among African American adolescents, for protective health messages.

In addition to the potential effects of differential targeting of health behaviors, family mores and norms necessarily play a role in the behaviors of these youth. As previously mentioned, the research shows that African American youth are more likely than other ethnic groups to use condoms (Grunbaum et al., 2002). This finding may possibly be connected to differing levels of communication about sexuality among African American parents and their children compared with Hispanics. There have been several studies that have examined the effectiveness of communication among African Americans in this context. A study among African American female adolescents suggested that communication about sexual matters among parents and their children, while not preventing engagement in sex, may result in more protective behaviors among adolescents (e.g., DiClemente, Wingood, Crosby, Cobb, Harrington, & Davies, 2001), and in a mixed gender African American sample, positive parental communication was correlated with increased condom use (Stanton, Li, Pack, Cottrell, Harris, & Burns, 2002).

Among Hispanic youth, however, communication about dangerous activities may not be the norm in households. VanOss Marin (2003) found for example, that talking about sex may generally be prohibited among Hispanics, and a focus group study among Latina women found a lack of agreement about discussions of sexuality with children (Talashek, Peragallo, Norr, & Dancy, 2004). Moreover, Ellickson and Morton (1999) found that poor communication with parents was a particularly important factor in the risk of drug use among a sample of Hispanic adolescents. These findings may help to explain the higher levels of unprotected sex while under the influence of substances among Cuban American adolescents in this sample.

Previous research has shown that risk factors play a differential role among different ethnic groups. For example, although more Black than White and Hispanic adolescents report easy access to hard drugs (e.g., cocaine, crack, heroin), fewer Blacks than Whites and Hispanics actually use hard drugs (SAMHSA, 2000). Turner and Lloyd (2003) found that lifetime cumulative exposure to adversity predicted risk of drug dependence. However, African American adolescents, who had significantly higher exposure to adversity than Cuban Americans, evidenced significantly lower lifetime rates of drug dependence disorder. The differential level of stressors, or perhaps the differential effects of the stressors, may offer an explanation for the varying levels of risky behaviors in the African American and Cuban American samples.

## *IMPLICATIONS FOR SOCIAL WORK PRACTICE*

The results of the current study have implications for (1) the development of interventions specifically targeted to incarcerated Cuban American and African American adolescents, and (2) the utilization of clinicians in these interventions. Incarceration may prove to be an advantage in delivering interventions while adolescents are temporarily accessible in confined settings (Magura, Shapiro, & Kang, 1994). In detention, barriers to risk reduction (e.g., substance use) are not present to interfere with program administration. Moreover, a specialized intervention with multiple training sessions can be implemented and long-term support and follow-up provided in the context of existing and re-entry programming. Studies which attempt to intervene with adolescents while they are detained have obtained some positive results such as increasing intentions and modifying attitudes towards using condoms with a new partner (e.g., Godin et al., 2003). As members of an interdisciplinary team, social workers could use their discipline specific skills to enhance such interventions within this context.

To improve the potential effectiveness of the prevention programs, interventions may need to include parental involvement as an important component, and address substance use issues in tandem with sexual behaviors, as research suggests that effectiveness may be limited otherwise (Castrucci & Martin, 2002; Otto-Salaj, Gore-Felton, McGarvey, & Canterbury, 2002). Integrating culturally specific components, for example, including staff persons who speak the target population's language and providing services in a culturally appropriate atmosphere, e.g., using culturally sensitive language and having respect for the values and beliefs of the target group, may improve the chances of program success (Medina & Johnson, 2004). Stuart (2004) suggests balancing the need to be respectful to cultural differences with the necessity for changing these beliefs as necessary. Sensitivity to cultural differences may also necessitate the acknowledgement that tensions exist among different ethnic groups and that group members of the same ethnicity prefer to interact only with each other. Clinicians may consider reducing potential conflicts by increasing interaction between the groups, confronting stereotypes and exploring differences and similarities to arrive at a consensus. The use of multicultural teams who can model effective teamwork/collaboration has also been suggested as a means of addressing the perceived tensions between groups (Morrison-Beedy, Carey, Aronowitz, Mkandawire, & Dyne, 2002).

For the interventions to be more effective, it would be important to include more than an educational component. The use of skills training, role plays to achieve mastery, and motivational enhancement for example, may improve the chances that the intervention will lead to reductions in unsafe sexual practices. Previous studies with samples of incarcerated and non-incarcerated youth showed that although overall knowledge of condoms and/or sexually transmitted risks was high, this knowledge was not correlated with positive attitudes or higher engagement in safer sexual behaviors (Morrison, Baker, & Gillmore, 1994; Shrier, Goodman, & Emans, 1999). Furthermore, it is extremely important that targeted efforts also address the environmental context in which these youth function because poor school systems, economic disadvantage, and community violence may neutralize the effects of positive influences (Kelly et al., 2003). Although this recommendation may be beyond the purview of an intervention for adolescents in detention, social workers may have a special role in providing community resource information, and in assisting with discharge planning and referrals to programs that provide positive influences for youth.

## REFERENCES

Blake, S.M., Ledsky, R., Goodenow, C., & O'Donnell, L. (2001). Recency of immigration, substance use, and sexual behavior among Massachusetts adolescents. *American Journal of Public Health, 91*, 794-798.

Castrucci, B.C., & Martin, S.L. (2002). The association between substance use and risky sexual behaviors among incarcerated adolescents. *Maternal and Child Health Journal, 6*, 43-47.

Centers for Disease Control and Prevention. (2002a). Fact Sheet–Young People at Risk: HIV/AIDS Among America's Youth. Retrieved December 2, 2003, from www.cdc.gov/hiv/pubs/facts/youth.htm.

Centers for Disease Control and Prevention. (2002b). HIV/AIDS among Hispanics in the United States. Retrieved March 22, 2004, from http://www.cdc.gov/hiv/pubs/facts/hispanic.htm.

Centers for Disease Control and Prevention. (2002c). HIV/AIDS Surveillance in Adolescents, L256 Slide Series (through 2001). Retrieved March 17, 2004, from www.cdc.gov/hiv/graphics/adolesnt.htm.

Centers for Disease Control and Prevention. (2002d). HIV and AIDS cases reported through December 2001. *HIV/AIDS Surveillance Report, 13*, 1-44.

DiClemente, R.J., Lanier, M.M., Horan, P.F., & Lodico, M. (1991). Comparison of AIDS knowledge, attitudes, and behaviors among incarcerated adolescents and a public school sample in San Francisco. *American Journal of Public Health, 81*, 628-630.

DiClemente, R.J., Wingood, G.M., Crosby, R., Cobb, B.K., Harrington, K., & Davies, S.L. (2001). Parent-adolescent communication and sexual risk behaviors among African American adolescent females. *Journal of Pediatrics, 139*, 407-412.

Ebin, V.J., Sneed, C.D., Morisky, D.E., Rotheram-Borus, M.J., Magnusson, A.M., & Malotte, C.K. (2001). Acculturation and interrelationships between problem and health promoting behaviors among Latino youth. *Journal of Adolescent Health, 28*, 62-72.

Ellickson, P.L., & Morton, S.C. (1999). Identifying adolescents at risk for hard drug use: Racial/ethnic variations. *Journal of Adolescent Health, 25*, 382-95.

Florida Annual Report/Epidemiologic Profile. (2002). Retrieved December 2, 2003, from www.doh.state.fl.us.

Gibson, D. R., & Young, M. (1994). Assessing the reliability and validity of self-reported risk behavior. In R. J. Battjes, Z. Slobada, & W. L. Grace (Eds.), *The context of HIV risk among drug users and their sexual partners.* (NIH Publication No. 94-3750, pp. 218-235). Rockville, MD: United States Department of Health and Human Services.

Godin, G., Michaud, F., Alary, M., Otis, J., Masse, B., Fortin, C., Gagnon, M., & Gagnon, H. (2003). Evaluation of an HIV and STD prevention program for adolescents in juvenile rehabilitation centers. *Health Education and Behavior, 30,* 601-614.

Grunbaum, J., Kann, L., Kinchen, S.A., Williams, B., Ross, J.G., Lowry, R., & Kolbe, L. (2002). Youth Risk Behavior Surveillance–United States, 2001. *In CDC Surveillance Summaries, Morbidity, and Mortality Weekly Report, 51,* 1-64.

Henry J. Kaiser Family Foundation. *The Tip of the Iceberg: The Global Impact of HIV/AIDS on Youth.* July 9, 2002. Fact Sheet #6043.

Jemmott, J.B., Jemmott, L.S., & Fong, G.T. (1992). Reductions in HIV risk-associated sexual behaviors among black male adolescents: Effects of an AIDS prevention intervention. *American Journal of Public Health, 82,* 372-377.

Kelly, P.J., Morgan-Kidd, J., Champion, J.D., & Wood, R. (2003). Sexuality knowledge, attitudes, and practices of young women in the juvenile justice system. *Pediatric Nursing, 29,* 271-277.

Khoury, E.L., Warheit, G.J., & Zimmerman, R.S. (1996). Gender differences in the prevalence of alcohol, cigarette, and illicit drug use over time in a multi-ethnic cohort of young adolescents in South Florida. *Women & Health,* 24, 21-40.

Magura, S., Shapiro, J.L., & Kang, S.Y. (1994). Condom use among criminally-involved adolescents. *AIDS Care, 6,* 595-603.

Malow, R.M, Devieux, J., Jennings, T.E., Lucenko, B. & Kalichman, S. (2001). Substance abusing adolescents at varying levels of HIV risk: Psychosocial characteristics, drug use and sexual behavior. *Journal of Substance Abuse,* 13, 103-117.

Medina, C., & Johnson, W. (2004). HIV/AIDS prevention in Latino and African-American communities. *Journal of the National Medical Association,* 96, 9S-11S.

Miller, K.S., Boyer, C.B., & Cotton, G. (2004). The STD and HIV epidemics in African American youth: Reconceptualizing approaches to risk reduction. *Journal of Black Psychology, 30,* 124-137.

Morrison, D.M., Baker, S.A., & Gillmore, M.R. (1994). Sexual risk behavior, knowledge, and condom use among adolescents in juvenile detention. *Journal of Youth and Adolescence, 23,* 271-288.

Morrison-Beedy, D., Carey, M.P., Aronowitz, T., Mkandawire, L., & Dyne, J. (2002). An HIV risk reduction intervention in an adolescent correctional facility: Lessons learned. *Applied Nursing Research, 15,* 97-101.

National Institute of Allergy & Infectious Diseases. (2002). HIV Infection in Adolescents: Fact Sheet. Rockville, MD: National Institutes of Health.

Otto-Salaj, L.L., Gore-Felton, C., McGarvey, E., & Canterbury, R.J. 2nd. (2002). Psychiatric functioning and substance use: Factors associated with HIV risk among incarcerated adolescents. *Child Psychiatry and Human Development, 33,* 91-106.

Otto-Salaj, L.L., Heckman, T.G., Stevenson, L.Y., & Kelly, J.A. (1998). Patterns, predictors, and gender differences in HIV risk among severely mentally ill men and women. *Community Mental Health Journal, 34*, 175-190.

Remez, L. (2000). Oral sex among adolescents: Is it sex or is it abstinence? *Family Planning Perspectives, 32*, 298-304.

SAMHSA. (2000). *Risk and protective factors for adolescent drug use: Findings from the 1997 National household survey on drug abuse.* Bethesda, MD: Substance Abuse and Mental Health Services Administration.

St. Lawrence, J.S., Crosby, R.A., & O'Bannon, R. III. (1999). Adolescent risk for HIV infection: Comparison of four high risk samples. *Journal of HIV/AIDS Prevention & Education for Adolescents & Children, 3*, 63-86.

Shrier, L.A., Goodman, E., & Emans, S.J. (1999). Partner condom use among adolescent girls with sexually transmitted diseases. *Journal of Adolescent Health, 24*, 357-61.

Sobell, L., Kwan, E., & Sobell, M. (1995). Reliability of a drug history questionnaire (DHQ). *Addictive Behavior, 20*, 233-241.

Sobell, L.C., & Sobell, M.B. (1980). Convergent validity: An approach to increasing confidence in treatment outcome conclusions with alcohol and drug abusers. In: L.C. Sobell, M.B. Sobell, & E. Ward (Eds.), *Evaluating Alcohol and Drug Abuse Treatment Effectiveness: Recent Advances,* pp. 177-183. New York: Pergamon Press.

Stanton, B., Li, X., Pack, R., Cottrell, L., Harris, C., & Burns, J.M. (2002). Longitudinal influence of perceptions of peer and parental factors on African American adolescent risk involvement. *Journal of Urban Health, 79*, 536-548.

Stuart, R.B. (2004). Twelve practical suggestions for achieving multicultural competence. *Professional Psychology: Research and Practice, 35*, 3-9.

Talashek, M.L., Peragallo, N., Norr, K., & Dancy, B.L. (2004). The context of risky behaviors for Latino youth. *Journal of Transcultural Nursing, 15*, 131-138.

Turner, R.J., & Lloyd, D.A. (2003). Cumulative adversity and drug dependence in young adults: Racial/ethnic contrasts. *Addiction, 98*, 305-315.

Unger, J.B., Cruz, T.B., Rohrbach, L.A., Ribisl, K.M., Baezconde-Garbanati, L., Chen, X., Trinidad, D.R., & Johnson, C.A. (2000). English language use as a risk factor for smoking initiation among Hispanic and Asian American adolescents: Evidence for mediation by tobacco-related beliefs and social norms. *Health Psychology, 19*, 403-410.

US Department of Justice (1999). *Minorities in the juvenile justice system. Juvenile Justice Bulletin: 1999 National Report Series,* Washington, DC, 1-16.

VanOss Marin, B.V. (2003). HIV prevention in the Hispanic community: Sex, culture, and empowerment. *Journal of Transcultural Nursing, 14,* 186-192.

Vega, W.A.,Gil, A.G., Warheit, G.J., Zimmerman, R.S., & Apospori, E. (1993). Acculturation and delinquent behavior among Cuban American adolescents: Toward an empirical model. *American Journal of Community Psychology, 21*, 113-125.

Vega, W.A., Gil, A.G., & Zimmerman, R.S. (1993). Patterns of drug use among Cuban-American, African-American, and white non-Hispanic boys. *American Journal of Public Health, 83*, 257-259.

# Acculturation Status and Substance Use Prevention with Mexican and Mexican-American Youth

Flavio F. Marsiglia
Stephen Kulis
David A. Wagstaff
Elvira Elek
David Dran

**SUMMARY.** This study examined whether language preference, as an indicator of acculturation, moderated the effects of a culturally grounded substance use prevention intervention for Mexican and Mexican American middle school students (N = 2,146) in Phoenix, Arizona. The main hypothesis was that levels of program effectiveness would vary based on

---

Flavio F. Marsiglia, PhD, is Associate Professor, Southwest Interdisciplinary Research Consortium, School of Social Work, Arizona State University, P.O. Box 873711, Tempe, AZ 85287-3711 (E-mail: marsiglia@asu.edu). Stephen Kulis, PhD, is Associate Professor and David Dran, MSW, is Graduate Associate, School of Social Work, SIRC, Arizona State University. David A. Wagstaff, PhD, and Elvira Elek, PhD, are Project Assistants, The Methodology Center, S153 Henderson, College of Health and Human Development, Pennsylvania State University.

This study was supported by National Institutes of Health/National Institute on Drug Abuse grants funding the Drug Resistance Strategies–The Next Generation Project (R01 DA14825) and the Southwest Interdisciplinary Research Consortium at Arizona State University (R24 DA13937).

[Haworth co-indexing entry note]: "Acculturation Status and Substance Use Prevention with Mexican and Mexican-American Youth." Marsiglia, Flavio F. et al. Co-published simultaneously in *Journal of Social Work Practice in the Addictions* (The Haworth Press, Inc.) Vol. 5, No. 1/2, 2005, pp. 85-111; and: *Substance Abusing Latinos: Current Research on Epidemiology, Prevention, and Treatment* (ed: Mario R. De La Rosa, Lori K. Holleran, and Shulamith Lala Ashenberg Straussner) The Haworth Press, Inc., 2005, pp. 85-111. Single or multiple copies of this article are available for a fee from The Haworth Document Delivery Service [1-800-HAWORTH, 9:00 a.m. - 5:00 p.m. (EST). E-mail address: docdelivery@haworthpress.com].

http://www.haworthpress.com/web/JSWPA

Digital Object Identifier: 10.1300/J160v05n01_05

the language preference of the students and the specific culturally grounded version of the intervention they were assigned. Findings show that matching language preference to particular versions of the intervention did not influence substance use related program outcomes, but that overall program effects (intervention versus control) did vary by language preference. English-language dominant participants, the most at risk sub-group, responded more positively to the intervention, while Spanish dominant, who had low substance use rates at baseline, and bilingual participants did not demonstrate significant differences between the intervention and control groups. Implications for school social work prevention interventions and prevention science in general, are discussed. 

**KEYWORDS.** Acculturation, substance abuse, protective factors, Mexican, Latino, youth, prevention

## *INTRODUCTION*

Studies show that the use of illicit drugs among teenagers in the United States declined significantly from 2001 to 2002, making 2002 the sixth year in a row such decreases have occurred (National Institute of Drug Abuse, 2003). Despite this encouraging news, differences in substance use among ethnic groups remain. African-American youth show substantially lower rates of overall use than Whites, while Latino youth show rates of use between these two other groups. However, for some regions of the country and for some substances, such as crack and ecstasy, Latino youth show the highest rates of use among all three groups (Johnston, O'Malley & Bachman, 2001). Rates of substance use for Latino youth may be depressed due to a school dropout rate much higher than that for African-Americans and Whites, since those who have left school before the 12th grade and not represented among survey respondents may be more at risk for substance use (Johnston et al., 2001). Substance use among Mexican and Mexican-American youth is especially troubling considering the growth of the Latino population, now approaching 13 percent of the U.S. population (Bureau of Census, 2000). In Phoenix, Arizona, where the present study was conducted, Latinos now constitute over one-third of residents, and the Latino population statewide grew from 1990 to 2000 at more than double the overall rate (U.S. Census, 2001).

While there has been increasing attention to ethnic differences in the delivery of prevention programs, few programs have been specifically grounded on the cultural characteristics of Mexican and Mexican-American youth (Polansky, Buki, Horan, Ceperich, & Burrows, 1999). Researchers have argued that prevention programs are more successful when they include elements of culture and ethnicity of the target population (Castro, Proescholdbell, Abeita, & Rodriguez, 1999). Although the importance of culturally appropriate messages in prevention efforts is increasingly acknowledged, tests of the effectiveness of such messages among minority cultures show mixed results. Supporting studies include those examining the effectiveness of television ads, where minority youth were more able to support messages when they could find in them reflections of their own culture (Dorr, 1982). Similar research has shown that youth and their parents respond more positively to drug prevention messages in the media that appear culturally specific (Teinowitz, 2001).

Prevention messages are considered culturally grounded when participants can recognize the messages as being about them and as applying to their lived experience (Marsiglia, Cross, & Mitchell, 1998). Questions remain regarding whether culturally grounded messages in prevention programs affect attitudes toward substance use, and whether the degree of cultural grounding influences the effectiveness of prevention interventions for Mexican American youth.

## *DEVELOPING CULTURALLY GROUNDED INTERVENTIONS*

Despite growing acceptance of the principle that prevention programs have a greater chance of participant acceptance when the interventions are compatible with their culture, the development of a truly culturally grounded approach to drug resistance can prove challenging. Often in an attempt to include culturally relevant material, programs may settle for untested or simplistic themes that may not in fact be culturally appropriate (Collins, 1995; Trimble, 1996). In addition to acknowledging sub-groups within larger umbrella cultural groups, such as Latinos/Hispanics or Asian Americans, research needs to recognize the heterogeneity existing within subgroups due to, among other factors, acculturation. If these factors are not considered, a program can run the risk of imposing stereotypical approaches, creating program content that does not resonate with the culture of the participants. In the prevention program that is the basis for the current study, The Drug Resistance Strategies Project, culturally grounded interventions were developed based on narratives of Phoenix, Arizona, middle school students regarding their situational encounters with drug offers and the students' refusal strategies (Hecht, Marsiglia, Elek, Wagstaff, Kulis, Dustman, & Miller-Day, 2003). Previous research affirmed that curriculum put in narrative form holds the attention of adolescent participants better than a simple discursive format (Botvin, Schinke, Epstein, & Diaz, 1994). The effort to cast the narratives into program curricula was informed by research which identified four major strategies of adolescents' drug resistance: Refuse, Explain, Avoid, and Leave (Miller-Rassulo, Alberts, Hecht, Krizek, & Trost, 2000). These strategies formed an acronym that students and project administrators used to coin the program: *keepin' it REAL* (*Manténte REAL* in Spanish).

Students from a high school in the same area as the participating middle schools were recruited to develop scripts and enact the scenarios from the narratives, which were then used to produce videotapes for the curriculum intervention in the study (Holleran, Dustman, Reeves, & Marsiglia, 2002). The videos included scenes from local neighborhoods that were readily identifiable by the study participants and were, at times, enacted by students known to the participants.

The resulting videos were an integral part of a ten session classroom curricula that was presented in three different versions. A Latino version represented scenarios from Mexican/Mexican American students, who formed a numerical majority in the participating schools. A non-Latino version of the curriculum contained scenarios derived from students who were African-American and European-American. These non-Latino students were in the numerical minority in all but a few of the participating schools. A third version of the curriculum combined an equal number of lessons and videos from each of the first two versions to form the Multicultural version (see Gosin, Marsiglia, & Hecht, 2003, and Holleran et al., 2002, for details on the curriculum and its development).

This study examines only the experiences of the Mexican and Mexican-American youth who took part in a larger study involving over 6,000 middle school students from an array of ethnic backgrounds. Previous analysis of outcomes for all participants in the randomized trial demonstrated the overall efficacy of the *keepin' it REAL* program in delaying or reducing substance use and in strengthening anti-drug norms and attitudes (Hecht et al., 2003). However, limited support emerged for the hypothesis that strictly matching the ethnicity of the students with the curriculum content significantly improves program outcomes, possibly because the students were so ethnically diverse as to raise questions about the degree of cultural match to particular program versions. Additional research on the efficacy of the intervention specifically for students of Mexican descent showed that, compared to controls, these students also demonstrated smaller increases in substance use and stronger anti-drug norms over time when participating in the two versions of the curriculum derived from their own cultural experience, the Latino and the Multicultural versions. This article further examines the efficaciousness of *keepin'it REAL* for Mexican origin students by considering how variations in acculturation status may have influenced both substance use outcomes and the effectiveness of the intervention.

## *ACCULTURATION AND SUBSTANCE USE*

Acculturation refers to individual-level as well as community-level changes in values, behaviors and preferred modes of expression that occur as a result of contact between two cultures (Berry, Poortinga, Segall, & Dasen, 1992). Especially for recent immigrants, acculturation involves a kind of socialization into mainstream conceptions of ethnicity and a reorientation that balances two conflicting needs–to preserve the culture of origin and yet become part of the new culture.

Research connecting acculturation to substance use has focused on protective social and personal factors that may stem from continued attachment to the culture of origin, and their weakening through acculturative processes that expose youth to risk behaviors through more acculturated peers, declining parental and family influence, and increasing acculturation-related stress. Aspects of traditional Mexican culture like *familism*, a cultural orientation that gives primacy to the family of origin even after marriage, have been associated with greater resilience to substance use. Mexican and Mexican-American families have been shown to have stronger family pride, family closeness and respect for parents, mutual obligation, trust, and cohesion than European American families (Chandler, Tsai, & Wharton, 1999). Traditional Mexican norms such as parental monitoring and involvement with children and the stress on geographic proximity of extended family members may also act protectively as they provide children with more attention from caring adults, and situate children in more cohesive communities (Chandler et al., 1999; Denner, 2001). On the other hand, migration can dislocate families and seriously limit their ability to rely upon relatives, *compadres* (ritualistic relatives) and friends (Menjivar, 2000; Patterson & Marsiglia, 2000). These protective aspects of culture can be weakened by acculturation and acculturation stress, resulting in greater vulnerability to substance use (De La Rosa, 2002).

Research has linked acculturation processes with higher levels of substance use as well as lowered educational aspirations for children of Mexican descent, both among immigrants and U.S.-born children (Samaniego & Gonzales, 1999; Vega & Gil, 1999). Language figures prominently in explanations for this connection. Some adolescents who are Spanish dominant appear sheltered from a developmentally driven expansion of their social networks that enables them to access the broader community and enter new situations where substances are offered, putting them at higher risk for substance use (Escobar, 1998; Gil and Wagner, 2000; Marsiglia & Waller, 2002; Marsiglia, Kulis, Hecht, & Sills, 2004). Because adults learn English more slowly than children do, acquisition of and preference for English by children in non-English proficient families can lead to an erosion of protective family ties and communication, and reinforce behaviors of the mainstream culture that cause value conflicts with the culture of origin (Marsiglia, Miles, Dustman, & Sills, 2002; Vega, Zimmerman, Warheit, Apospori, & Gil, 1997).

## *PREFERRED LANGUAGE AS AN INDICATOR OF ACCULTURATION*

Acculturation can be a difficult concept to measure and one that needs to be approached multi-dimensionally (Weigers & Sherraden, 2001). Much of the existing research and scale development on acculturation has focused on adults. The challenge in addressing the comparative lack of valid and reliable measures of acculturation for children and adolescents is to recognize the complexity of acculturation while at the same time considering youths' ethnic identity development (Serrano & Anderson, 2003; Unger, Gallaher, Shakib, Ritt-Olson, Palmer, & Johnson, 2002). In the absence of developmentally appropriate measures that assess acculturation across affective, behavioral, and cognitive domains, generation status and language use continue to be the most commonly used measures of acculturation. Although preferred language has been criticized as an oversimplified measure of acculturation, it has been demonstrated to be a good proxy for more sophisticated and multi-dimensional measures, accounting for up to 65% of the variance on acculturation status (Rogler et al., 1991; Samaniego & Gonzales, 1999). Language use measures have also been useful in alerting us to the existence of acculturation stress and the subsequent presence of substance use (Cuellar, Arnold, & Maldonado, 1995). Recent mediational research predicting Latino adolescents' substance use has employed measures of "linguistic acculturation" based on preferred language use (Epstein, Doyle, & Botvin, 2003).

Language preference continues to enter into investigations of substance use. Recent household surveys of alcohol use across several groups of Latino youth–Cuban, Mexican-American, Puerto Rican, South American and Central American–showed little difference among the various Latino groups, but large and consistent differences in alcohol use across all groups by language use. The more respondents used English language, the more likely they were to drink alcohol (Nielsen & Ford, 2001). Similarly, students using Spanish at home reported significantly less marijuana use than students who speak English with their parents (Epstein, Botvin, & Díaz, 2001), and bilingual Hispanic youth were found at greater risk of alcohol use than Spanish monolingual youth (Epstein, Botvin, & Díaz, 2000). A study conducted with Mexican-American middle school students in the Southwest found that students who spoke only Spanish used significantly less alcohol and other drugs than bilingual students or students who preferred to use English (Marsiglia & Waller, 2002).

The relationship between acculturation, ethnic self-identity, and substance use for youth is consistently highlighted by the specialized literature, but the multi-faceted impacts of acculturation and ethnic identity on substance use are just beginning to be understood. One way that a drug prevention program might be effective with this population is by slowing the erosion of traditional Mexican cultural norms regarding the family and drug involvement. Through a process called additive acculturation, culturally grounded and multicultural interventions may help children deal with acculturation issues by encouraging successful integration into the new culture without losing the identity-enhancing and protective aspects of the old culture (Gibson, 1995). The present study aims at advancing knowledge about the impact of acculturation on the efficacy of the *keepin' it REAL* substance use prevention program for a sample of Mexican and Mexican-American youth in the Southwest borderlands region.

## *HYPOTHESES OF THE STUDY*

This study examines whether language preference, as a proxy for acculturation, moderates the effects of *keepin'it REAL* among Mexican and Mexican-American youth. It tests for differences in program effects between more and less acculturated students, generally expecting that those who are more acculturated will be more "at-risk" of onset of substance use and therefore more likely to show desired program effects.

> *H1*: Desired program outcomes, as indicated by relatively less substance use and stronger anti-drug norms in intervention groups compared to control groups, will be stronger among English dominant than among bilingual and Spanish dominant students.

In addition, we expect that the different versions of the *keepin' it REAL* curriculum will be differentially effective for students in different acculturation statuses. If so, program outcomes will be influenced by interaction effects between language preference, as a proxy for acculturation, and curriculum version.

> *H2a*: Spanish dominant students will report less substance use and stronger anti-drug norms when participating in the Latino version than in the Multicultural or Non-Latino versions of the curriculum.
> *H2b*: Bilingual students will report less substance use and stronger anti-drug norms when participating in the Multicultural than in the Latino or Non-Latino curriculum versions.
> *H2c*: English dominant students will demonstrate less substance use and stronger anti-drug norms when participating in the non-Latino than in the Multicultural or Latino versions of the curriculum.

## *METHOD*

### *Research Design*

The present study employed a pretest-posttest experimental design with three intervention conditions and one control condition. Self-report data were collected at the two time periods from students enrolled in 35 public middle schools in the central corridor of the Phoenix metropolitan area. The schools were stratified by size of enrollment and ethnicity (% Latino) and then randomly assigned to one of four conditions-Latino, Non-Latino, Multicultural, or Control–with 8 to 10 schools in each condition. In Fall 1998, all 7th graders in the study schools were administered a baseline or pretest questionnaire. In Spring 1999, their regular 7th grade classroom teachers delivered the assigned curriculum version to intervention students. During that summer, a bilingual radio/television PSA and billboard campaign was fielded. During the following school year (1999-2000), the intervention schools implemented school-based booster activities with their 8th grade students. Finally, in Spring 2000, approximately 14 months after completing the classroom-based curriculum in the intervention schools, a posttest questionnaire was administered to all 8th grade students who were then enrolled in the 35 study schools, including some students who had not completed the pretest. During the period that elapsed between the pretest and posttest, students in the control condition participated in the existing substance use prevention programs chosen and instituted by their school or school district personnel to meet state mandates for prevention programming (see Hecht et al., 2003, for more detailed information).

### *Participants*

The reported findings are based on data provided by 2,146 students in the study schools who completed the pretest questionnaire during 7th grade and/or the posttest questionnaire in 8th grade and reported their race/ethnicity solely as "Mexican American, Mexican, or Chicano." This sample was 52% male. Over three-quarters of the study schools had majority Latino enrollments, overwhelmingly comprised of students of Mexican descent.

### *Questionnaires*

The questionnaires (each up to 82 items) utilized a three-form design (Graham, Hofer, & MacKinon, 1996) that employed planned missingness to limit the number of questionnaire items each individual student answered, while maximizing the total number of items included for analysis. Project-trained proctors rather than regular teachers administered the 45-minute questionnaires that were printed in English on one side and in Spanish on the other side. The questionnaires were completed during regular school hours, typically in science, health, or homeroom classes. Students were given written and verbal guarantees of confidentiality, and told that their participation was voluntary.

## *MEASURES*

### *Demographic Characteristics*

The questionnaires identified the Mexican descent students through six yes or no items that asked if they were: (a) Mexican American, Mexican, Chicano/a; (b) Other Latino (Puerto Rican, Cuban, etc.); (c) White (Anglo); (d) African American (Black); (e) American Indian (Pima, Yaqui, Navajo, etc.); or (f) Asian or Pacific Islander (Chinese, Japanese, etc.). Students could report mixed ethnic backgrounds. The current analysis is restricted to those who only marked "yes" to the first item at baseline or at posttest. Students reported their gender by marking male or female, their age by indicating their birth date, and their federal school lunch participation (a proxy for socioeconomic status) by selecting whether or not they received a free or reduced price school lunch.

### *Acculturation Status*

The students' preferred language was used as a proxy measure for acculturation. Students who indicated they spoke "Spanish only" or "Spanish mostly" with friends, as well as those who opted to complete the posttest questionnaire in Spanish were assigned to the "Spanish dominant" group. Of the remaining students, those who indicated they spoke "both English and Spanish, about equal" with friends were assigned to a "Bilingual" group; and students indicating they spoke "mostly" or "only" English with friends were assigned to the "English dominant" group. Table 1 shows the breakdown of the participating students by their language preference and study condition.

### *Substance Use Outcomes*

The questionnaire included self-reports of how much and how frequently students drank alcohol, smoked cigarettes, and smoked marijuana in the past 30 days. Up to 95% agreement has been reported

TABLE 1. Language Preference by Condition Breakdown of Mexican and Mexican American Respondents

| Language Preference | Condition: Latino Version | Non-Latino Version | Multicultural Version | Control |
|---|---|---|---|---|
| Spanish | 15% (70) | 22% (88) | 26% (161) | 21% (142) |
| Bilingual | 39% (181) | 32% (126) | 37% (229) | 36% (241) |
| English | 46% (213) | 45% (178) | 38% (235) | 42% (282) |
| Total | 100% (464) | 100% (392) | 100% (625) | 100% (665) |

*NOTE:* The proportion of students indicating each language preference differs significantly by condition ($\chi^2 = 22.75$, $df = 6$, $p < .01$) with a somewhat smaller proportion of Spanish preference in the Latino condition, and a larger proportion of Spanish preference in the Multicultural condition.

between saliva samples and drug use self-reports (Ellickson and Bell, 1990). Evidence supporting the validity of self-report data is especially strong when, as in the current study, analyzing reports on drug use activities during the last 30 days (O'Malley, Bachman, & Johnston, 1983; Johnston, 1989), and comparing self-reports over time and across treatments (Smith-Donals & Klitzner, 1985). The study's substance use items were modeled after Likert scales used by Flannery, Williams, & Vazsonyi (1999) with a similar age population. To assess the amount, students indicated number of drinks (1 = *None* to 9 = *More than 30*), cigarettes (1 = *None* to 8 = *More than two packs*), and hits of marijuana (1 = *None* to 8 = *More than 40*). Frequency of each of the three types of substance use was measured in terms of the number of days of use in the last month (1 = *None* to 6 = *16 to 30*). The responses on amount and frequency were averaged, both separately for each substance as well as all together across substances to obtain an additional measure of overall recent substance use, which demonstrated high internal consistency (Cronbach's $\alpha = .86$).

### *Refusal Confidence*

This three-item measure assessed students' confidence (1 = *Not at all sure* to 5 = *Very sure*) in saying no to alcohol, tobacco, and other drug offers from "a friend (they) really liked," "someone (they) don't know well," or "a family member (parents, brothers, sisters, aunts, uncles, etc.)." The measure was based on Kasen, Vaughan, and Walter's (1992) self-efficacy scale, and was formed by averaging the three item scores; larger scores indicated greater confidence in ability to refuse drug offers. Internal consistency (α) was .74.

### *Intentions to Accept Substance Use Offers*

This measure assessed intentions to accept hypothetical offers of "alcohol to drink (beer, wine, hard liquor)," "a cigarette," or "marijuana" (1 = *Definitely no* to 4 = *Definitely yes*). The three item scores were averaged; larger scores indicated stronger intentions to accept offers. Internal consistency (α) was .81.

### *Positive Substance Use Expectancies*

This six-item measure assessed students' perceptions of the positive consequences of substance use. Three alcohol items (Hansen & Graham, 1991) asked if drinking alcohol makes it easier "to be part of a group," "to have a good time with friends," or "makes parties more fun." Two cigarette items asked if "smoking cigarettes makes people less nervous" and if smoking makes "it easier to concentrate." One item asked if smoking marijuana makes "food taste better." The response choices for all six items, scored from 1 (*Never*) to 5 (*Most of the time*), were averaged to form a scale score; larger scores indicated more positive substance use expectancies. Internal consistency (α) was .74.

### *Personal, Injunctive, and Descriptive Norms*

The Focus Theory of Norms (Cialdini, Kallgren & Reno,1990) guided the selection of measures of three distinctive types of drug related norms: personal (what the individual thinks is right or wrong), injunctive (what the individual believes that others think is right or wrong) and descriptive (how many of their peers use drugs). Based on Likert items used by Hansen and Graham (1991), anti-drug personal norms were assessed by asking: "Is it OK for someone your age to . . ." "drink alcohol," "smoke cigarettes," or "use marijuana." Possible responses ranged from 1 (*Definitely OK*) to 4 = (*Definitely Not OK*). The three item personal norms measure demonstrated high internal consistency of α = .86. The items related to anti-drug injunctive norms focused on important reference groups for youth (parents and best friends) and were based on those used by Hansen and Graham (1991) and

Hansen, Johnson, Flay, Graham, and Sobel (1988). The items asked how angry students' parent(s) would be if they found out that the student "smoked marijuana," "smoked cigarettes," or "drank alcohol" (three individual items scaled 1 = *Not angry at all* to 4 = *Very angry*), and how their best friends would react if they engaged in these actions (three additional items on scales of 1 = *Very friendly* to 4 = *Very unfriendly*). Internal consistency (α) was .71 and .81 respectively for the parent injunctive norms and best friend injunctive norms measures. Lastly, to assess descriptive norms, two items asked the respondents to estimate how many students in their schools had tried alcohol, tobacco, and other drugs at least once, and how many students in their schools use drugs regularly (both on scales of 1 = *Hardly any* to 4 = *Most*; α = .72).

### *Variables Used Only for Missing Data Imputation*

Multiple imputations was used to handle missing data. In addition to the variables above, the imputation model included measures of current grades (1 = *Mostly F's* through 9 = *Mostly A's*), and how far the students expected to get in school (1 = *Finish 8th grade* through 5 = *Finish 4 years of college*).

## *STATISTICAL ANALYSES*

The analysis proceeded in three stages. To address the planned missingness and the missing data due to wave and item non-response, the software package NORM (Schafer, 1997; Schafer & Olsen, 1998) was used to generate ten multiply imputed data sets. To preserve potential interaction effects with study condition, the imputations were performed separately for each of the four conditions of the randomized design (three versions of the intervention, one control). Next, for each imputed data set, students' change scores on given outcomes were regressed on baseline scores and a dummy variable for study condition (e.g., for comparisons of the intervention versions, we regressed the change score on students' baseline scores and two dummy-coded intervention version variables). Thus, the dependent variable is a change score adjusted for baseline differences. This model is equivalent to an analysis of covariance on posttest scores (see Huitema, 1987). In this second stage, adjusted mean differences among study condition groups and the variance of each mean difference were written to a data file. Finally, Carlin, Li, Greenwood, and Coffey's (2002) implementation of Rubin's rules (1987) was used to combine the ten sets of estimates and test the hypothesis that the mean change reported by certain study condition students equaled that reported by comparison students.

All of the analysis models accounted for school-level randomization with the accompanying nesting of students within school. With group assignment to a study condition, responses of students from the same school are expected to be more similar to each other than are the responses of any two students chosen at random. The number of participants from the 35 study schools (i.e., the cluster size) ranged from 30 to 460, with Latino students being the majority group in over three-fourths of the schools. Each of the analysis models tested four sets of variables with simultaneous regression models. These sets consisted of (a) overall substance use; (b) separate alcohol, cigarette, and marijuana use; (c) personal, descriptive, and parents' and friends' injunctive norms; and (d) refusal confidence, intentions to accept substance use offers, and positive expectancies about substance use.

The first analysis model compared outcomes among different versions of the curriculum with each other and did not include the control group. Additionally, this model tested for the main effects of acculturation status (Spanish, bilingual, or English language preference, with English as the omitted reference group) and the interaction of intervention version by language preference. A second analysis model was used to compare the three versions of the intervention combined together against the control condition, and assess the interaction of language preference with whether or not the student received the intervention. The third analysis model examined the intervention versus control difference separately for Spanish dominant, bilingual, and English dominant students.

## *RESULTS*

### *Interaction of Language Preference and Version of the Intervention*

The first model (see Table 2) used dummy coding to contrast the three intervention versions, test the language preference main effect, and test the interaction between intervention version and language preference. The dummy variables permitted a test for adjusted mean differences associated with two of the intervention versions (Latino and non-Latino), two of the language preference groups (Spanish and bilin-

TABLE 2. Main Effects of Intervention Version and Language Preferences and the Interaction Effects of Language Preference and Version of the Intervention on Substance Use and Substance Use Related Outcomes

| | Intervention Version versus Grand Mean | | Language Preference versus Grand Mean | | Interaction | Covariate |
|---|---|---|---|---|---|---|
| Outcome Variables | Latino Version | Non-Latino Version | Spanish Dominant | Bilingual | Intervention Version X Language Preference[a] | Baseline (W1) Value |
| | Est./SE | Est./SE | Est./SE | Est./SE | Est./SE | Est./SE |
| Overall Substance Use | −.01/.06 | .00/.08 | −.04/.05 | −.03/.04 | NS | −.42/.06*** |
| Alcohol Use | .02/.10 | .03/.13 | −.04/.08 | −.04/.08 | NS | −.56/.05*** |
| Cigarette Use | −.02/.06 | −.04/.06 | .01/.05 | −.03/.04 | NS | −.69/.05*** |
| Marijuana Use | −.05/.08 | .04/.10 | −.11/.06 | −.02/.05 | NS | −.39/.06*** |
| Refusal Confidence | .04/.07 | −.06/.08 | .14/.05** | .00/.05 | NS | −.65/.04*** |
| Intentions to Accept | −.04/.05 | .00/.05 | −.08/.04* | −.01/.02 | NS | −.58/.03*** |
| Positive Expectancies | .01/.06 | .00/.05 | −.12/.05* | .01/.03 | NS | −.53/.03*** |
| Personal Anti-Drug Norms | .05/.06 | −.04/.06 | .05/.03 | .00/.03 | NS | −.61/.04*** |
| Parents' Injunctive Norms | .07/.05 | −.08/.05 | .00/.04 | .02/.03 | NS | −.56/.06*** |
| Friends' Injunctive Norms | .04/.06 | .00/.05 | .18/.04*** | −.03/.03 | NS | −.58/.05*** |
| Descriptive Norms | −.09/.08 | .01/.08 | −.03/.04 | .01/.03 | NS | −.71/.03*** |

[a] Represents four specific dummy variable interaction contrasts: Spanish dominant and in Latino version (Y/N); bilingual and in Latino version (Y/N); Spanish dominant and in Non-Latino version (Y/N); bilingual and in non-Latino version (Y/N) .
NS indicates non-significant at $p < .05$, $^{*}p < .05$, $^{**}p < .01$, $^{***}p < .001$.

gual) and their four multiplicative interaction terms. The reference group in these comparisons is English dominant students in the Multicultural version of the intervention. The tests of the interaction effects explicitly examine the primary hypotheses that acculturation, as assessed by language preference, moderates the effects of particular versions of the intervention. Any such effects would support the idea of matching the version of the intervention to the language preference of the students. This analysis was limited to the 1,481 intervention students; it excluded students in the control condition since it was concerned only with which version of the intervention worked best for students of a given language preference (i.e., it compared the versions to each other and not to the control group).

Table 2 reports main and interaction effects of intervention version and language preference on eleven substance use related outcomes. Results show that the three intervention versions did not differ significantly from one another in predicting posttest outcomes when controlling for language preference and baseline differences on those outcomes. In addition, as none of the interaction contrasts were statistically different from 0, there was no support for the interaction between intervention version and language preference. However, there were some significant differences associated with language preference as a main effect, showing more desirable outcomes for Spanish dominant students. Table 3 illustrates the nature and direction of these effects more clearly by reporting mean differences from baseline to posttest for students in each language preference category, and separately for intervention students (all versions combined) and controls. Specifically, among the intervention students, refusal confidence and friend's injunctive norms increased more, intentions to accept substance use offers increased less, and positive expec-

TABLE 3. Unadjusted Mean Difference and Standard Errors from Pre-Intervention to 14-Month Follow-Up for the Intervention Versions Together and the Control Condition by Language Preference

| | Intervention Condition | | | Control Condition | | |
|---|---|---|---|---|---|---|
| | Spanish Dominant | Bilingual | English Dominant | Spanish Dominant | Bilingual | English Dominant |
| | Est./SE | Est./SE | Est./SE | Est./SE | Est./SE | Est./SE |
| Recent Substance Use | .18/.07 | .15/.06 | .18/.07 | .10/.07 | .29/.09 | .53/.08 |
| Alcohol | .28/.10 | .22/.09 | .27/.10 | .19/.14 | .43/.10 | .66/.16 |
| Cigarettes | .12/.07 | .04/.05 | .06/.06 | .00/.07 | .14/.09 | .26/.09 |
| Marijuana | .14/.09 | .19/.07 | .23/.08 | .10/.09 | .28/.13 | .66/.13 |
| Refusal Confidence | .22/.11 | .14/.07 | .01/.08 | .04/.13 | .03/.11 | −.30/.10 |
| Intent to Accept | .08/.05 | .12/.04 | .12/.04 | .02/.08 | .15/.08 | .31/.05 |
| Positive Expectancies | −.09/.07 | .00/.05 | .05/.06 | −.01/.11 | .06/.10 | .22/.06 |
| Norms | | | | | | |
| Personal Anti-drug | −.07/.07 | −.08/.06 | −.05/.05 | .01/.08 | −.16/.10 | −.32/.06 |
| Parents' Injunctive | −.03/.05 | −.04/.05 | −.06/.05 | −.03/.08 | −.06/.05 | −.11/.05 |
| Friends' Injunctive | .05/.06 | −.12/.05 | −.14/.06 | .05/.11 | −.25/.08 | −.29/.07 |
| Descriptive | .31/.08 | .10/.09 | .02/.06 | .24/.10 | .18/.08 | .29/.08 |

tancies of substance use decreased more for Spanish language dominant students than for English dominant and bilingual students. Because similar patterns could also be observed among the control students, we examined the main effect of language preference further in analyses that included both intervention and control students.

## *INTERACTION OF LANGUAGE PREFERENCE AND RECEPTION OF THE INTERVENTION*

The second model, like the first model, used dummy coding to examine the main effects of the intervention (with control students included in the sample and used as the reference group), the main effects of language preference, and the interaction of the intervention with language preference. This model collapsed the three versions of the intervention into one intervention group because analyses of the first model indicated no significant differences in program outcomes among the different versions of the intervention. The tests of the interaction effects explicitly examined whether acculturation, as assessed by language preference, moderated the effects of the intervention, i.e., whether the intervention appeared more beneficial for students of one language preference than for students of another language preference group. In summary, dummy coding permitted us to estimate and test in models the adjusted mean differences associated with the intervention effect, two of the language preference groups (Spanish and bilingual), and two contrast interaction terms formed by multiplying the dummies for condition and language preference. This particular set of analyses included all 2,146 students (see Table 4).

As shown by Table 4, when controlling for language preference and baseline differences, the intervention only affected positive substance use expectancies. There was a significant main effect for language preference for most outcomes, following the pattern of differences in Table 3. Overall substance use, alcohol use, marijuana use, intentions to accept substances, positive expectancies of substance use, and descriptive norms, all increased less for Spanish language dominant students than for English dominant and bilingual students. Refusal confidence, personal anti-drug norms, and friend's anti-drug injunctive norms on average all decreased less for the Spanish dominant students than for the English dominant and bilingual students. On the other hand, the bilingual students did not demonstrate significantly different outcomes from the Spanish and English dominant students. In contrast to the model

TABLE 4. Main Effects of Intervention and Language Preference and the Interaction Effects of Language Preference and Reception of the Intervention on Substance Use and Substance Use Related Outcomes

| | | Language Preference versus Grand Mean | | Interaction | Covariate |
|---|---|---|---|---|---|
| Variables | Intervention versus Control | Spanish Dominant | Bilingual | Intervention X Language Preference[a] | Baseline (W1) Value |
| | Est./SE | Est./SE | Est./SE | Est./SE | Est./SE |
| Overall Substance Use | −.06/.03 | −.14/.04** | −.02/.03 | .10/.04* & −.01/.03 | −.39/.05*** |
| Alcohol Use | −.07/.05 | −.17/.06** | −.01/.05 | .12/.06 & −.02/.05 | −.53/.04*** |
| Cigarette Use | −.02/.03 | −.06/.04 | −.02/.03 | .07/.04 & .00/.03 | −.63/.05*** |
| Marijuana Use | −.07/.04 | −.20/.06** | −.04/.04 | .09/.05 & .02/.04 | −.39/.05*** |
| Refusal Confidence | .09/.04 | .15/.05** | .04/.04 | −.02/.04 & −.03/.04 | −.63/.03*** |
| Intentions to Accept | −.02/.02 | −.14/.03*** | −.01/.02 | .06/.03* & .00/.02 | −.57/.02*** |
| Positive Expectancies | −.05/.03* | −.13/.04** | −.01/.03 | .02/.04 & .01/.03 | −.52/.03*** |
| Norms | | | | | |
| Personal Anti-Drug | .04/.03 | .13/.03*** | .00/.03 | −.07/.03* & .00/.03 | −.64/.03*** |
| Parent's Injunctive | .02/.03 | .02/.03 | .02/.02 | −.02/.03 & .00/.02 | −.56/.04*** |
| Friend's Injunctive | .06/.03 | .23/.04*** | −.04/.03 | −.05/.03 & .01/.03 | −.56/.04*** |
| Descriptive | −.03/.03 | −.11/.04** | .03/.03 | .09/.03* & −.02/.03 | −.70/.03*** |

[a] Two dummy variable estimates and standard error are presented in this column, the first for Spanish dominant Intervention students (Y/N) and the second for Bilingual Intervention students (Y/N).
*$p < .05$, **$p < .01$, ***$p < .001$.

which looked at language preference within intervention version, this model, which compared the three versions combined together to the control, did produce significant interaction effects on some of the outcomes, specifically overall substance use, intentions to accept substance use offers, personal anti-drug norms, and descriptive norms. Students reporting different levels of language preference reacted to the intervention differently on some of the outcomes. This supported further testing of some related simple effects to better describe what was going on with the interventions.

As shown by Table 4, when controlling for language preference and baseline differences, the intervention only affected positive substance use expectancies. There was a significant main effect for language preference for most outcomes, following the pattern of differences in Table 3. Overall substance use, alcohol use, marijuana use, intentions to accept substances, positive expectancies of substance use, and descriptive norms, all increased less for Spanish language dominant students than for English dominant and bilingual students. Refusal confidence, personal anti-drug norms, and friend's anti-drug injunctive norms on average all decreased less for the Spanish dominant students than for the English dominant and bilingual students. On the other hand, the bilingual students did not demonstrate significantly different outcomes from the Spanish and English dominant students. In contrast to the model which looked at language preference within intervention version, this model, which compared the three versions combined together to the control, did produce significant interaction effects on some of the outcomes, specifically overall substance use, intentions to accept substance use offers, personal anti-drug norms, and descriptive norms. Students reporting different levels of language preference reacted to the intervention differently on some of the outcomes. This supported further testing of some related simple effects to better describe what was going on with the interventions.

### *Examination of Interaction Effects*

A third model made extensive use of single-degree-of-freedom contrasts to compare the three intervention versions combined together to the control within each language preference group, as well as to contrast program outcomes for the English language dominant students with those of the Spanish dominant and the bilingual students (see Table 5). This particular set of analyses included all 2,146 students.

Table 5 shows the results of the analyses utilizing this covariate-adjusted model. The intervention demonstrated significant effects only for the English language dominant students. These effects reflect the appreciable pretest to posttest changes in undesirable directions for most outcomes that were exhibited by the English dominant students in the control group, those who preferred to speak English with their friends, and completed the questionnaire in English (see Table 3). In comparison, English dominant students in the intervention condition reported significantly smaller increases in overall substance use, recent cigarette use, recent marijuana use, intentions to accept substance use offers, positive substance use expectancies, and descriptive norms. The intervention clearly appeared to be of some value to the English dominant students. The lack of significant differences between the intervention and control conditions for the other two language preference groups

TABLE 5. Comparison of Intervention to Control Within Each Language Preference Group, Along with Comparisons of Among Language Preference Groups on Substance Use and Substance Use Related Outcomes

| | Intervention versus Control Simple Effects Test Within Language Preference | | | Spanish Dominant or Bilingual vs. English Dominant | English Dominant or Spanish Dominant vs. Bilingual | Covariat |
|---|---|---|---|---|---|---|
| Outcome Variables | Spanish Dominant | Bilingual | English Dominant | | | Baseline (W1) Value |
| | Est./SE | Est./SE | Est./SE | Est./SE | Est./SE | Est./SE |
| Overall Substance Use | .04/.04 | −.06/.05 | −.15/.05** | −.16/.04*** | .02/.03 | −.39/.04*** |
| Alcohol Use | .04/.07 | −.10/.06 | −.16/.09 | −.18/.06** | .01/.05 | −.53/.04*** |
| Cigarette Use | .04/.04 | −.03/.04 | −.09/.05* | −.08/.04* | .02/.03 | −.63/.05*** |
| Marijuana Use | .02/.05 | −.05/.06 | −.18/.08* | −.24/.05*** | .04/.04 | −.43/.04*** |
| Refusal Confidence | .07/.07 | .05/.05 | .14/.05* | .19/.04*** | −.04/.04 | −.63/.03*** |
| Intentions to Accept | .04/.03 | −.02/.03 | −.09/.03** | −.15/.02*** | .01/.02 | −.57/.02*** |
| Positive Expectancies | −.04/.05 | −.04/.04 | −.08/.04* | −.14/.03*** | .01/.03 | −.52/.03*** |
| Norms | | | | | | |
| Personal Anti-Drug | −.04/.04 | .04/.04 | .11/.04** | .13/.03*** | .00/.03 | −.64/.03*** |
| Parent's Injunctive | −.01/.04 | .02/.03 | .04/.03 | .03/.02 | −.02/.02 | −.56/.04*** |
| Friend's Injunctive | .00/.05 | .07/.04 | .10/.05 | .19/.04*** | .05/.03 | −.56/.04*** |
| Descriptive | .06/.05 | −.06/.04 | −.10/.04* | −.08/.03** | −.03/.03 | −.70/.03*** |

*$p < .05$, **$p < .01$, ***$p < .001$.

provides some evidence that a lack of acculturation may be acting as a protective factor for the Spanish dominant (and possibly bilingual) students. In other words, in the absence of the intervention, Spanish dominant students would not move in undesirable directions on the substance use related variables as much as English dominant students would. Therefore the intervention does not appear effective for them because there is less of a problematic substance use trajectory to influence. In fact, a comparison of the English dominant students to the Spanish dominant and bilingual students in the study (Table 5, column 4) demonstrated significantly worse outcomes for the former on each of the outcomes, except for parental anti-drug injunctive norms.

The elevated risk associated with acculturation appeared in baseline mean scores showing that English dominant students actually reported the highest rates of substance use and intentions to accept substance use offers, the most positive expectancies of substance use, and the weakest anti-drug personal norms and friend injunctive norms at the outset of the study (see Table 6). The Spanish dominant students reported the lowest rates of substance use and intentions to accept substance use offers, the strongest refusal confidence, the least positive expectancies of substance use, and the strongest anti-drug friend and personal norms and perceived that fewer of their peers were experimenting with or using substances regularly at the outset of the study.

## *DISCUSSION*

Overall, youth of Mexican descent who participated in the program showed more favorable outcomes in substance use and in attitudes toward drug use than their counterparts in the control condition. This study demonstrated that identification and use of culturally grounded drug prevention interventions for middle school students is feasible and can have an impact on the use of substances by Mexican and Mexican-American youth. Participants who preferred to speak Spanish used substances less at both the beginning and at the end of the intervention

TABLE 6. Unadjusted Baseline Means for the Intervention (Combined) and Control Conditions by Language Preference

| | Intervention Condition | | | Control Condition | | |
|---|---|---|---|---|---|---|
| Outcome Variable | Spanish Dominant | Bilingual | English Dominant | Spanish Dominant | Bilingual | English Dominant |
| | Est./SE | Est./SE | Est./SE | Est./SE | Est./SE | Est./SE |
| Recent Substance Use | 1.37/.07 | 1.47/.06 | 1.63/.07 | 1.40/.07 | 1.46/.11 | 1.53/.06 |
| Alcohol | 1.57/.09 | 1.73/.08 | 1.87/.09 | 1.58/.10 | 1.69/.13 | 1.75/.10 |
| Cigarettes | 1.25/.06 | 1.33/.05 | 1.37/.03 | 1.31/.07 | 1.26/.09 | 1.33/.06 |
| Marijuana | 1.29/.08 | 1.36/.07 | 1.68/.09 | 1.28/.10 | 1.42/.15 | 1.51/.07 |
| Refusal Confidence | 3.64/.08 | 3.56/.07 | 3.56/.08 | 3.72/.12 | 3.57/.08 | 3.61/.08 |
| Intent to Accept | 1.62/.04 | 1.67/.04 | 1.83/.05 | 1.56/.07 | 1.70/.07 | 1.81/.05 |
| Positive Expectancies | 2.09/.06 | 2.15/.06 | 2.24/.06 | 2.07/.10 | 2.20/.12 | 2.24/.07 |
| Norms | | | | | | |
| Personal Anti-Drug | 3.42/.05 | 3.35/.05 | 3.22/.04 | 3.42/.09 | 3.35/.10 | 3.28/.06 |
| Parents' Injunctive | 3.45/.05 | 3.50/.04 | 3.48/.03 | 3.47/.07 | 3.48/.05 | 3.44/.06 |
| Friends' Injunctive | 3.00/.06 | 2.92/.05 | 2.75/.06 | 2.99/.10 | 2.92/.09 | 2.67/.07 |
| Descriptive | 2.21/.08 | 2.55/.10 | 2.69/.07 | 2.16/.07 | 2.60/.07 | 2.57/.07 |

compared to participants who preferred to speak English, confirming that Spanish language preference serves as a protective factor against substance use for this population (Epstein, Doyle, & Botvin, 2003; Marsiglia & Waller, 2002). However, English dominant Mexican and Mexican-American participants, considered the most at risk, demonstrated more desirable outcomes across the intervention groups than their counterparts in the control condition. Mexican and Mexican-American youth participating in this study demonstrated significantly more favorable outcomes in any version of the curriculum than their counterparts in the control group.

No support was found, however, for the hypothesis that program outcomes would be moderated by particular matches between intervention version and language preference. Specifically, we expected that English dominant, bilingual, and Spanish dominant students would show stronger desired program effects, respectively, in the Non-Latino, Multicultural and Latino versions of the intervention. The lack of support for matching language preference to program version can be the result of the very low use rate self-reported by Spanish dominant students at baseline. However, English dominant participants demonstrated the strongest desired program effects for both substance use and attitudes toward substance use after participation in any version of the curriculum. The program was able to reach these youth who have been identified in several studies as most at risk of substance use involvement (Epstein, Botvin, & Diaz, 2000; 2001).

This study employed language preference as an unsophisticated proxy for acculturation. It is recognized that acculturation is a multidimensional concept that is not adequately captured in a simple measure of language preference. However, this proxy for acculturation has some advantages. Language preference has been found to account for a substantial portion of variance in the development of more detailed scales for acculturation (Cuéllar, Harris, & Jasso, 1980; Marin & Marin 1991). Language preference is a critical part of students' moves from more to less sheltered social contexts. It captures important elements in acculturation models that allow for competence in more than one culture under different circumstances (Coleman et al., 2001). Such a view of acculturation would fit the experience of Mexican and Mexican-American youth who–through English language acquisition–find their social horizons widening beyond their family and same culture friends. A culturally grounded intervention may have a favorable effect for Mexican and Mexican-American youth who would be exposed increasingly to drug offers and opportunities to use substances that come with a broadening social landscape and new friendship networks disconnected from culture of origin and family control. A multicultural intervention may also provide skills in drug refusal not only for situations taken from Mexican and Mexican-American cultures, but also for drug offer scenarios originating from European-American and African-American peer groups.

It appears that Spanish language as an indicator of lower levels of acculturation has a protective effect against the risk of adolescent substance use. To delay intervention until these protective effects are eroded by higher acculturation may jeopardize the goal of primary prevention. School-based, culturally grounded interventions such as *keepin'it REAL* appear to serve well Mexican/Mexican-American students throughout the acculturation continuum. The lack of significant effects on Spanish monolingual students can be traced to their baseline low or non-existent substance use rates. In order to better estimate the impact of this intervention or similar universal interventions researchers face the challenge of developing and testing alternative measures to the traditional drug use behavioral based measures. Survey data should provide longitudinal profiles of students as they progress through their acculturation process based on multi measure survey instruments. A lack of significance between baseline and posttest over 14 months may be speaking of an adequate interval for assessing change among students who are initially at low risk, particularly those who are still early adolescents and Spanish dominant. These students, if neglected by prevention interventions, may quickly lose the protective effects of culture of origin and join their substance-using peers.

These findings have important implications for school social workers, other school-based prevention professionals, and for prevention research in general. When is the right time to intervene? Are Spanish monolingual Mexican descent students protected by culture of origin, and if so, do they need to be exposed to a substance use prevention curriculum? Should resources target bilingual and English dominant Mexican-American students more heavily? Answers to the questions must await further research into the dynamics of acculturation and acculturation stress processes.

School social workers can play a key role as cultural mediators between school and home, between majority cultural norms and culture of origin. In the borderlands as in other regions of the nation, social workers can support students of immigrant background to celebrate their cultural heritage and family and stay connected to their protective effects. Students need the support of social workers as they navigate through multiple transitions. They are not just adolescents but they also need to negotiate at least two cultures and two languages as they develop a sense of self. Racism, xenophobia, and a relentless and generalized push toward complete language and cultural assimilation can be a source of great stress and may lead to self-medication. Social workers can intervene early and through science based programs support our youth to stay in school, to stay healthy, and to be proud of their families and their cultural heritage.

## REFERENCES

Berry, J.W., Poortinga, Y.H., Segall, M.H., & Dasen, P.R. (1992). *Cross-cultural psychology: Research and applications.* New York: Cambridge University Press.

Botvin, G.J., Schinke, S.P., Epstein, J.A., & Diaz, T. (1994). Effectiveness of culturally focused and generic skills training approaches to alcohol and drug abuse prevention among minority youths. *Psychology of Addictive Behaviors*, 8, 116-127.

Carlin, J.B., Li, N., Greenwood, P., & Coffey, C. ( 2002). Tools for analyzing multiple imputed data sets. Preprint of a manuscript submitted to *The Stata Journal.*

Castro, F. G., Proescholdbell, R.J., Abeita, L., & Rodriguez, D. (1999). Ethnic and cultural minority groups. In B.S. McCrady & E.E. Epstein (Eds.), *Addictions: A comprehensive guidebook* (pp. 499-526). New York: Oxford Press.

Chandler, C.R., Tsai, T.M., & Wharton, R. (1999). Twenty years after: Replicating a study of Anglo- and Mexican-American cultural values. *The Social Science Journal*, 36, 2, 353-367.

Cialdini, R., Reno, R., & Kallgren, C. (1990). A focus theory of normative conduct: Recycling the concept of norms of reduce littering in public places. *Journal of Personality and Social Psychology*, 58, 6, 1015-1026.

Coleman, H.L.K., Casali, S.B., Wampold, B.E., (2001). Adolescent strategies for coping with cultural diversity. *Journal of Counseling and Development*, 79, 356-364.

Collins, R.L. (1995). Issues of ethnicity in research on prevention of substance abuse. In G.J. Botvin, S. Schinke, & M.A. Orlandi (Eds.), *Drug abuse prevention with multiethnic youth* (pp. 28-45). Thousand Oaks, CA: Sage.

Cuéllar, I., Arnold, B., & Maldonado, R. (1995). Acculturation Rating Scale for Mexican Americans-II: A revision of the original ARSMA scale. *Hispanic Journal of Behavioral Sciences*, 17, 275-304.

Cuéllar, I., Harris, L.C. & Jasso, R. (1980). An acculturation scale for Mexican-American normal and clinical populations. *Hispanic Journal of Behavioral Science*, 2, 199-217.

De La Rosa, M. (2002). Acculturation and Latino adolescents' substance use: A research agenda for the future. *Substance Use and Misuse*, 37, 4, 429-456.

Denner, J., Kirby, D., & Coyle, K. (2001). The protective role of social capital and cultural norms in Latino communities: A study of adolescent births. *Hispanic Journal of Behavioral Sciences,* 23, 1, 3-21.

Dorr, A. (1982). Television and the socialization of the minority child. In G.I. Mitchell-Kernan & C. Mitchell-Kernan (Eds.), *Television and the socialization of the minority child* (pp. 15-36). New York: Academic Press.

Ellickson, P.L., & Bell, R.M. (1990). Drug prevention in junior high: A multi-site longitudinal test. *Science*, 247, 1299-1305.

Epstein, J.A., Botvin, G.I., Diaz, T. (2000). Alcohol use among Hispanic adolescents: Role of linguistic acculturation and gender, *Journal of Alcohol and Drug Education* 45, 18-32.

Epstein J.A., Botvin, G.I., Diaz T. (2001). Linguistic acculturation associated with higher marijuana and polydrug use among Hispanic adolescents. *Substance Use and Misuse*, 6, 4, 477-499.

Epstein, J.A., Doyle, M., Botvin, G.J. (2003). A mediational model of the relationship between linguistic acculturation and polydrug use among Hispanic adolescents. *Psychological Reports*, 93, 3, 859-866.

Escobar, J.I. (1998). Immigration and mental health: Why are immigrants better off? *Archives of General Psychiatry*, 55, 9, 781-782.

Flannery, D.J., Williams, L.L., & Vazsonyi, A.T. (1999). Who are they with and what are they doing? Delinquent behavior, substance use, and early adolescents' after-school time. *American Journal of Orthopsychiatry*, 69, 247-253.

Gibson, M.A. (1995). Additive acculturation as a strategy for school improvement. In R.G. Rumbaut and W.A. Cornelius (Eds.), *California's immigrant children: Theory, research and implications for educational policy* (pp. 77-105). San Diego: Center for U.S.-Mexican Studies, University of California.

Gil, A.G., & Wagner, E.F. (2000). Acculturation, familism, and alcohol use among Latino adolescent males: Longitudinal relations. *Journal of Community Psychology*, 28, 443-458.

Gosin, M., Marsiglia, F.F., & Hecht, M.L. (2003). *Keepin' it REAL*: A drug resistance curriculum tailored to the strengths and needs of pre-adolescents. *Journal of Drug Education*. 33, 2, 119-142.

Graham, J.W., Hofer, S.M., & MacKinon, D.P. (1996). Maximizing the usefulness of data obtained with planned missing value patterns: An application of maximum likelihood procedures. *Multivariate Behavioral Research*, 31, 197-218.

Hansen, W.B., & Graham, J.W. (1991). Preventing alcohol, marijuana, and cigarette use among adolescents: Peer pressure resistance training versus establishing conservative norms. *Preventive Medicine*, 20, 414-430.

Hansen, W.B., Johnson, C.A., Flay, B.R., Graham, J.W., & Sobel, J. (1988). Affective and social influence approaches to the prevention of multiple substance abuse among seventh grade students: Results from Project SMART. *Preventive Medicine*, 17, 135-154.

Hecht, M.L., Marsiglia, F.F., Elek, E., Wagstaff, D., Kulis, S., Dustman, P., & Day, M. (2003). Culturally-grounded substance use prevention: An evaluation of the *keepin' it R.E.A.L.* curriculum. *Prevention Science*, 4, 4, 233-248.

Holleran, L., Dustman, P., Reeves, L., & Marsiglia, F. F. (2002). Creating culturally grounded videos for substance abuse prevention: A dual perspective on process. *Journal of Social Work Practice in the Addictions*, 2, 1, 55-78.

Huitema, B.E. (1987). *The analysis of covariance and alternatives*. New York, NY: John Wiley & Sons, Inc.

Johnston, L.D. (1989). The survey technique in drug abuse assessment. *Bulletin on Narcotics, 41*, 29-39.

Johnston, L.D., O'Malley, P.M., & Bachman, J.G. (2001). The Monitoring the Future National survey results on adolescent drug use: Overview of key findings, 2000 (NIH Publication No. 01-4923). Bethesda, MD: National Institute on Drug Abuse, c. 56 pp.

Kasen, S., Vaughan, R.D., & Walter, H.J. (1992). Self-efficacy for AIDS preventive behaviors among 10th grade students. *Health Education Quarterly*, 9, 187-202.

Marin, G., Marin, B.V. (1991) *Research with Hispanic Populations: Applied Social Research Methods Series*, Volume 23. Newberry Park, CA: Sage Publications.

Marsiglia, F.F., Cross, S. & Mitchell, V. (1998). Culturally grounded group work with adolescent American Indian students. *Social Work with Groups*, 21, 1/2, 89-102.

Marsiglia, F.F., Kulis, S., and Hecht, M. (2001). Ethnic labels and ethnic identity as predictors of drug use among middle school students in the Southwest. *Journal of Research on Adolescence*, 11, 1, 21-48.

Marsiglia, F.F., Miles, B.W., Dustman, P. A. & Sills, S. K. (2002). Ties that protect: An ecological view of protective factors influencing urban adolescent substance use. *Journal of Ethnic and Cultural Diversity in Social Work*, 11, 3/4, 191-220.

Marsiglia, F.F., & Waller, M. (2002) Language preference and drug use among Southwestern Mexican-American middle school students, *Social Work in Education*, 24, 3, 145-158.

Marsiglia, F.F., Kulis, S., Hecht, M.L., & Sills, S. (2004). Ethnicity and ethnic identity as predictors of drug norms and drug use among pre-adolescents in the Southwest. *Substance Use & Misuse, 39*, 7, 1061-1094.

Menjivar, Cecilia. 2000. *Fragmented Ties: Salvadoran Immigrant Networks in America.* Berkeley: University of California Press.

Miller-Rassulo, M., Alberts, J.K., Hecht, M.L., Krizek, R.L., & Trost, M. (2000). *Adolescent Relationships and Drug Abuse.* NY: Erlbaum Publications.

National Institute of Drug Abuse. (2003). NIDA Notes, Research News. Vol. 17, 5, retrieved from the World Wide Web *http://www.drugabuse.gov/NIDA_notes/NNVol17N5/Teen.html* on Friday, March 14, 2003

Nielsen, A., & Ford, J.A., (2001). Drinking patterns among Hispanic adolescents: Results from a national household survey. *Journal of Studies on Alcohol,* 62, 448ff.

O'Malley, P.M., Bachman, J.G., & Johnston, L.D. (1983). Reliability and consistency in self-reports of drug use. *The International Journal of the Addictions*, 18, 806-824.

Patterson, S., & Marsiglia, F.F. (2000). 'Mi casa es su casa': A beginning exploration of Mexican Americans' natural helping. *Families in Society*, 81, 1, 22-31.

Polansky, J.M., Buki, L.P., Horan, J.J., Ceperich, S.D., Burows, D.D. (1999). the effectiveness of substance abuse prevention videotapes with Mexican-American adolescents. *Hispanic Journal of Behavioral Sciences*, 21, 186-198.

Rubin, D.B. (1987). *Multiple imputation for nonresponse in surveys.* New York, NY: John Wiley.

Samaniego, R.Y., & Gonzales, N.A. (1999). Multiple mediators of the effects of acculturation status on delinquency for Mexican American adolescents. *American Journal of Community Psychology*, 27, 2, 189-210.

Schafer, J.L. (1997). *Analysis of Incomplete Multivariate Data.* New York: Chapman and Hall.

Schafer, J.L., & Olsen, M.K. (1998). Multiple imputations for multivariate missing data problems: A data analyst's perspective. *Multivariate Behavioral Research*, 33, 545-571.

Serrano, E., & Anderson, J. (2003). Assessment of a refined short acculturation scale for Latino preteens in rural Colorado. *Hispanic Journal of Behavioral Sciences*, 25, 2, 240-253.

Smith-Donals, L., & Klitzner, M. (1985). Self-reports of youthful drinking and driving: Sensitivity analyses of sensitive data. *Journal of Psychoactive Drugs*, 17, 179-190.

Teinowitz, I. (2001). Anti-drug messages should send ethnic adults distinct culture cues. *Advertising Age*, 72, 14.

Trimble, J.E. (1996). Alcohol abuse in urban adolescents and women: A longitudinal study for assessment and risk evaluation. *American Indian and Alaska Native Mental Health Research,* 7, 81-90.

Unger, J.B., Gallaher, P., Shakib, S., Ritt-Olson, A., Palmer, P.H., & Johnson, C.A. (2002). The AHIMSA acculturation scale: A new measure of acculturation for adolescents in a multicultural society. *Journal of Early Adolescence*, 22, 3, 225-251.

U.S. Census 2000. (2001). retrieved December 30, 2001 from the World Wide Web: *http://azcentral.com/news/census/census.html/.*

U.S. Census Bureau. (2000). Overview of race and Hispanic origin, [online] retrieved December 30, 2001 from the World Wide Web: *http://www.census.gov/population/cen2000/briefs.html/*

Weigers, M., & Sherraden, M. (2001). A critical examination of acculturation: The impact of health behaviors, social support, and economic resources on birth weight among women of Mexican descent, *International Migration Review*, 35, 804-839.

Vega, W.A., & Gil, A.G. (1999). A Model for explaining drug use behavior among Hispanic adolescents. *Drugs & Society*, 14, 57-74.

Vega, W.A., Zimmerman, R.S., Warheit, G.J., Apospori, E., & Gil, A.G. (1997). Acculturation strain theory: Its application in explaining drug use behavior among Cuban and other Hispanic youth. *Substance Use & Misuse*, 32, 12-13, 1943-1948.

# Culturally Competent Intervention with Families of Latino Youth at Risk for Drug Abuse

Dhira Crunkilton
Juan J. Paz
David P. Boyle

**SUMMARY.** A culturally specific intervention for families with children at risk for substance abuse was implemented by *Proyecto Juventud* (Youth Project), a community-based family services program located in the rural southwestern United States. This intervention, incorporating culturally appropriate language, beliefs, values, and principles, provided substance abuse education to families. Participants were pretested at intake and posttested at one year, utilizing one measure for knowledge of drugs and drug abuse, and a second measure for family functioning. Results indicated that parents' scores relating to drug and drug abuse knowledge showed a trend of improvement on 16 out of 20 items. The results on family functioning were inconclusive. The study illustrated

---

Dhira Crunkilton, MSW, is a doctoral candidate, University of Georgia. Juan J. Paz, DSW, is Associate Professor, Arizona State University. David P. Boyle, LCSW, PhD, is Director of Studies in Social Work, Division of Social Sciences, Dalton State College.

Address correspondence to: Dhira Crunkilton, 310 East Campus Drive, School of Social Work, University of Georgia, Athens, GA 30602 (E-mail: dcrunkil@uga.edu).

[Haworth co-indexing entry note]: "Culturally Competent Intervention with Families of Latino Youth at Risk for Drug Use." Crunkilton, Dhira, Juan J. Paz, and David P. Boyle. Co-published simultaneously in *Journal of Social Work Practice in the Addictions* (The Haworth Press, Inc.) Vol. 5, No. 1/2, 2005, pp. 113-131; and: *Substance Abusing Latinos: Current Research on Epidemiology, Prevention, and Treatment* (ed: Mario R. De La Rosa, Lori K. Holleran, and Shulamith Lala Ashenberg Straussner) The Haworth Press, Inc., 2005, pp. 113-131. Single or multiple copies of this article are available for a fee from The Haworth Document Delivery Service [1-800-HAWORTH, 9:00 a.m. - 5:00 p.m. (EST). E-mail address: docdelivery@haworthpress.com].

http://www.haworthpress.com/web/JSWPA

Digital Object Identifier: 10.1300/J160v05n01_06

the importance of using a cultural approach with Latino families in the area of substance abuse prevention. 

**KEYWORDS.** Latino substance abuse prevention, family intervention, culturally specific intervention

## *INTRODUCTION*

Research on Latino parental influences consistently points to the critical role that the attitudes and behaviors of parents play in predicting early use of substances by their children (Coombs, Paulson, & Richardson, 1991; Department of Health and Human Services, 1995; Hawkins, Catalano, & Miller, 1992; Hernandez & Lucero, 1996; Johnson & Johnson, 1999; Scheier, Botvin, & Miller, 1999; Sealy, 2000; Vega, Kourney, Zimmerman, & Gil, 1995). Researchers have emphasized that adolescent support networks may be more important in explaining drug use behavior than the individual characteristics of the adolescents themselves (Krohn & Thornberry, 1993; Wallace, 1999). Latino parental influence and quality of the parent-child relationship were critical predictors in the initiation and experimentation of alcohol, tobacco, and other drug use among high-risk youth (Coombs et al., 1991; Hawkins et al., 1992).

Recent studies (Scheier et al., 1999; Sealy, 2000) further emphasized the key importance of the parent-child relationship in substance abuse prevention. Sealy's evidence revealed that the higher the level of parental support, as defined as praise, encouragement, and physical affection, the less often the adolescent drank alcohol. Scheier et al. found that the beneficial life experiences of Hispanic youth such as "family communication," as well as an internal health focus of control, buffered the effects of negative life events on alcohol use. Johnson and Johnson (1999) also reported on the buffering effect of the Hispanic family on the initiation of alcohol use by children and adolescents. In a press release summarizing a critical juncture in the accumulation of research pointing to the importance of parent-child communication in light of increasing rates of Latino youth drug use, Chavez (1999) stated:

> As the Substance Abuse and Mental Health Services Administration National Household Survey on Drug Abuse has shown, heavy alcohol use among Hispanic/Latino youth has doubled in the last few years. And following all trends of youth, there has been an increase of illicit drug use among Hispanic/Latino youth during the 1990s . . . Research shows that parents are consistently identified by young people as the most important trustworthy sources of information and guidance on substance abuse and other serious issues . . . We know that parents, grandparents, foster parents, and other caring adults can play a major role in helping young people avoid substance abuse . . . the key is talking with our children often and early. (p. 1)

Latino parents' alcohol and drug use behaviors have also been studied as predictors of their children's alcohol and drug use behaviors. Geroerer and De La Rosa (1993) reported a relationship between Latino parents' illicit drug use and children's use. Barrera Jr. and Li (1993) noted the presence of alcoholism/problem drinking in Latino parents tended to correlate with elevated drinking among their adolescent children. Studies on the relationship between substance abuse of parents and subsequent alcohol problems in their children were reviewed by J. L. Johnson and Leff (1999), and additional research (Barrera Jr. & Li, 1995; Barrera Jr., Li, & Chassin, 1998; Gilbert, Solis, & Mora, 1992) suggested that ethnicity and alcoholism in parents were factors influencing the stress of adolescents.

In addition to issues of poor family relationships and parental drug use, some Latino youth are subjected to other factors which may place him or her at risk for drug abuse. Additional risk factors include the influence of friends and social networks, acculturation stressors such as culture shock, intergenerational and acculturation gaps, language barriers, and identity conflicts (Rhodes & Jason, 1990; Szapocznik et al., 1989). Vega et al. (1995) discussed the issue that some Hispanic adolescents feel themselves caught between family and cultural values and the dominant society's expectations. Some adolescents may turn to substance abuse as one of many coping mechanisms.

Figueroa-Moseley (1998) reported that the degree of acculturation of Latino adolescents was associated with the likelihood of substance abuse; however, individuals who were bicultural or had medium acculturation were at the greatest risk for substance abuse. Another study (Perez & Padilla, 2000) concluded that within a few generations, most Hispanic adolescents exhibited a predominant American culture orientation while maintaining some traces of their Hispanic cultural orientation. Although home culture orientation diminished across generations, it did not disappear completely; many adolescents retained allegiance to their Hispanic familial values. These findings suggest that the Latino child's cultural orientation or degree of acculturation is important to assess when considering substance abuse prevention.

The main idea underlying a culturally sensitive intervention is that adolescents from different ethnic backgrounds are exposed to a different set of risk factors, requiring culturally relevant methodologies and programs. Culturally based approaches in relation to Latino family issues including substance abuse have been frequently addressed in the literature (Austin & Pollard, 1993; Delgado, 1998a; Flores & Carey, 2000; Gilbert et al., 1992; Glick & Moore, 1990; Kar, 1999; Krestan, 2000; Maddahian, Newcomb, & Bentler, 1988; Mayers, Kail, & Watts, 1993; Sotomayor, 1991; Szapocznik, Amaro, & U.S. Dept. of Health and Human Services, 1995; Vega & Gil, 1998; Vega et al., 1995). In their study of cultural conflicts and problem behaviors of Latino adolescents in home and school environments, Vega et al. reported a connection between the parent-adolescent relationship and alcohol use. Their findings alerted professionals to the necessity of designing interventions to include family and culture. Researchers (Acosta & Hamel, 1995; Delgado, 1995, 1996) have recommended that practitioners also recognize natural support systems as an important ingredient of Hispanic culture and integrate the natural support system into all aspects of alcohol and other drug services practice with this population.

Another issue to consider in planning a comprehensive intervention is Latino family functioning. Sokol-Katz and Ulbrich (1992) were interested in family functioning in terms of the structure of the family. They examined whether family structure, as defined by which or both parents were present, was related to alcohol and drug use among Mexican, Puerto Rican, and Cuban American adolescents. Mexican adolescents living in female-headed households had higher rates of drinking, drug use, and overall risk-taking behaviors (RTBs) than those living with both parents. By comparison, Puerto Rican adolescents living in female-headed households had higher rates of overall RTBs than those living with both parents. In the Cuban adolescent group, family structure was unrelated to RTBs. Figueroa-Moseley (1998) also studied the relationship of Hispanic family structure and the likelihood of substance abuse in children; however, these findings were inconclusive.

The current study did not examine family structure, but did consider detailed patterns in family functioning. The necessity to include factors of both family functioning and culture in prevention models for Latino youth has been emphasized in previous studies (Rhodes & Jason, 1990; Szapocznik et al., 1989). Santisteban, Szapocznick, and Rio (1993) presented an overview of conceptual models and practical approaches in working with Latino youth already identified as alcohol and other drug (AOD) users, as well as those considered at high risk for future AOD use, and discussed the role of the family in the behavior problem syndrome. Researchers have made literature available for scientists, decision makers, and service providers to develop a deeper understanding of the role families and culture play in the prevention of alcohol and other drug abuse in Hispanic/Latino American populations (Department of Health and Human Services, 1995). Issues in preventing alcohol and other drug abuse among Hispanic/Latino families, as well as issues of behavior problems among Hispanic/Latino youth have been explored (Department of Health and Human Services). Family-based intervention models have been implemented and tested in high-density Hispanic/Latino communities throughout the United States and Puerto Rico (Delgado, 1998b; Department of Health and Human Services, 1995).

An example of a comprehensive urban prevention program including variables of family and culture was *La Familia* (Hernandez & Lucero, 1996). *La Familia*'s community-based alcohol, tobacco, and other drug (ATOD) prevention program targeted Latino families with high-risk youth age from age 6 to 11. *La Familia* attempted to reduce identified risk factors while building on culturally relevant protective factors. During a two year period, the program enrolled over 200 youth and their families through existing community networks and aggressive outreach; Hernandez and Lucero reported a 92% retention rate and over 80% attendance per session. As a result of the program, families became more willing to discuss ATOD issues openly.

Based on the similar vital features of family, culture, and community, the current study proposed a family intervention as part of a comprehensive rural community-based program called *Proyecto Juventud* (Youth Project). *Proyecto Juventud* was aimed at meeting the prevention needs of rural Latino youth demonstrating high-risk characteristics for substance abuse. Like *La Familia, Proyecto Juventud* proposed a specific intervention to increase family participation, which would hopefully lead to open discussion of ATOD issues.

## METHOD

### Design and Sample

This study incorporated a pre-experimental pretest posttest group design. The family intervention was part of a larger program, which included an intervention for youth. Participants in the family intervention were selected when their child was randomly chosen for participation in the youth intervention. The sampling frame for the youth intervention was created by several community agencies cognizant of children at risk of substance abuse, in a rural area of the southwest United States. After children were randomly selected from the list, parents were contacted. The nature of the program was explained to the parents, and they were asked to sign a consent form in either English or Spanish, in which they gave consent for their child's participation. Parents who gave consent for their child to participate created the selection pool for this study. Forty-nine parents representing 49 different families made up the sample by self-selection. Parents were assured that their participation was confidential.

This study tested two hypotheses:

1. Families in the community who participate in the culturally competent intervention *Proyecto Juventud* will improve their scores on family functioning as measured by the FACES III.
2. Families in the community who participate in the culturally competent intervention *Proyecto Juventud* will improve their scores on measures of drug knowledge.

The independent variable is the "service offered to families who participate in a culturally competent intervention." The two dependent variables are "scores on family functioning" and "scores on drug use knowledge."

### Measures

The Family Profile Questionnaire was designed by the program evaluator to generate both descriptive and experimental data. The level of acculturation was measured by the Acculturation Rating Scale for Mexican Americans-ASRMA II (Cuellar, Arnold, & Maldonado, 1995). The ARSMA II, totaling 48 items, consisted of a Mexican Orientation Scale and an Anglo Orientation Scale. ARSMA II has two subscales,

Anglo Orientation (AOS) and Mexican Orientation (MOS). Both subscales have good internal reliabilities, with Cronbach's alpha = .86 and .88 for the AOS and MOS, respectively. ARSMA II appears to have good face validity, and has been demonstrated to have strong construct validity (Cuellar, Arnold, & Maldonado).

Two instruments, the Family Adaptability and Cohesion Evaluation Scale (FACES-III), and a drug knowledge questionnaire were used to generate the experimental data for testing the two hypotheses.

The Family Adaptability and Cohesion Evaluation Scale, or the FACES III (Olsen, 1986) has become the benchmark measuring instrument for family functioning (McClanahan, 1998). The history preceding the development of FACES III goes back to the Timberlawn Institute in Dallas, Texas, which was the first organization to produce such research on variables of family functioning (Lewis, Beavers, Gosset, & Phillips, 1976). The institute initiated development of rating scales to measure dimensions of family functioning such as structural organization, power, individuation, expression, and how members deal with separation (Lewis et al.).

FACES III (Olsen, 1986) measures three family qualities: cohesion, adaptability, and family type. *Cohesion,* measured by 10 questions using a Likert-type scale, deals with the parents' perception of how cohesive they and their children are, as a group. *Adaptability*, also measured by 10 items using a Likert-type scale, deals with the parent's perception of how adaptable they and their children are, as a group. These two scores are combined and averaged, to calculate a *Family type*, which indicates the degree of healthy balance.

FACES III has total instrument alpha of .68, which is considered fair internal consistency (Olsen as cited in Fischer & Corcoran, 1994). The subscales' internal consistency scores are .77 for cohesion, and .62 for adaptability. Five week test-retest correlation was reported to be .83 for cohesion and .80 for adaptability. FACES III appears to have good face validity, and a number of studies have shown that the previous version, FACES II, had fair known-groups validity. FACES III has been tested on 2.453 adults and 412 adolescents (Fischer & Corcoran).

The drug knowledge questionnaire consisted of 20 "true or false" questions referring to a range of substances, including cigarettes (nicotine), alcohol, marijuana, inhalants, barbiturates, and cocaine. The test appears to have good face validity. An example of an item about cigarettes was "Smoking cigarettes is harmful to the unborn child." An example related to cocaine was "Regular cocaine inhalation rarely causes addiction."

### *Data Collection*

The supervising agency for *Proyecto Juventud* employed bi-lingual social workers to collect data. Workers were trained in the basic techniques of administering questionnaires, including instruction in confidentiality, maintaining neutrality, preserving the integrity of the data, and the time frame for the study. The pretest Family Profile Questionnaire was administered to the parents during the first family camp. The questionnaires were again administered to the parents at the final family camp approximately 12 months later, for the posttest.

### *Intervention*

The intervention was carried out by a team of social workers who were assisted by volunteers via two main strategies. One strategy was family camps (*campamentos*) and the other was family support groups (*pláticas familiares*). The intervention, including culturally appropriate themes, focused on activities designed to involve parents in learning about substance abuse prevention, to support family functioning, and to increase the families' protective factors. The educational components of the entire intervention included: (a) tobacco use, (b) HIV/AIDS, (c) alcohol, (d) other drugs, (e) drug related domestic violence, (f) parent/child relationships and (g) teacher/parent relationships.

### *Family Camps*

Ten *family camps* in the year were held at various sites. The length of each *family camp* varied according to the site. Indoors *camps* were held in the local community; these lasted a few hours in the evenings or on a weekend day. Outdoor *family camps,* requiring travel and camping for a duration of two to four days, were held at southwest state and national parks, such as the Grand Canyon, Mogollon Rim, Canyon de Chelly, Sedona, and Catalina. *Family camps* were designed to provide the youth and their parents the opportunity to get away from their usual home setting which allowed for an arena facilitating more open discussion. For the camping trips, all families were invited to attend and supplied camping equipment. Families who chose to attend then traveled by car caravan, led by staff, to a family camping site which had been pre-arranged by the staff. After arriving at the site, families and staff proceeded with camping activities: setting up the camp, preparing meals, and participating in recreational activities such as hiking, swimming, games, and nightly campfires. In addition to these activities, interactions were structured to give both parents and their children opportunities to discuss issues related to alcohol, tobacco, and other drugs (ATOD) and to work on the families' issues such as decision making and problem solving. Another focus was on how families could develop proactive healthy lifestyles to enhance their protective factors. Often, these discussions occurred during campfire talks, as well as part of skits that were performed.

### *Family Support Groups*

Held every three to four weeks in their community, family support groups met for a total of 13 meetings in the year. The support groups lasted 3.5 hours. Churches and homes were utilized for locations of the support groups. It was believed that support groups held in a setting that is familiar to families would promote participation. The topics included basic information about ATOD use and abuse, as well as problem solving techniques and mutual support.

## *DATA ANALYSIS AND RESULTS*

Data collected by the evaluation team was processed using the Statistical Package for the Social Sciences (SPSS, Version 10.0). Descriptive statistics were calculated to determine demographics, drug use, and acculturation. An independent sample t-test was conducted to determine whether there were significant differences between the mean scores for the pretests and the posttests of the FACES III. Descriptive statistics were also compiled for the pretest and posttest of the drug knowledge inventory.

### *Participant Characteristics*

A total of 49 parents were interviewed at pretest. Each of the parents had one or more children participating in the project. The average parent age was 38.7 with a range of 27 to 65 years of age. The breakdown of ethnicity was as follows: 39 Mexican Americans or 79%; 7 African Americans, or 14%; 2 Native Americans, or 5%; and 1 White, or 2%. The mean number of children per household under age 18 was 3.5. The mean parent education was a ninth grade education. All the respondents were female. Over half, 53%, were married, 14.3% were divorced, 16.3% were separated, 14.3% were single, and 2% were widowed.

### *Acculturation*

The ARSMA II was used to assess orientation to Mexican or American cultures. Item scores range from one to five, with one being a more Mexican orientation and five being a more Anglo orientation. Results indicated that parents who participated had a mean score of 1.9, indicating a strong Mexican orientation.

### *Self-Reported Drug Use*

Response to 12 questions assessed the parents' self-reported use of ATOD (N = 49). Table 1 displays the actual percentages of affirmative responses on each question.

Almost 57% of the parents reported that they had tried alcohol, while 26.1% reported use in the last month. Almost 44% of parents reported trying cigarettes, and 28.3% reported using cigarettes in the last month. While almost 11% acknowledged that they had tried marijuana, 2.2% admitted that they had used marijuana in the last month. When asked about cocaine and other drugs, 2.2% of the parents reported that they had tried each. For the past month use, no one reported using cocaine, but 2.2% responded that they had used "other drugs." Considering inhalants, parents said they had neither tried nor used this substance.

TABLE 1. Percent of Parents Reporting Having Tried Substance, and Reporting Last Month Use (N = 49)

| Substance | Percent of parents who had ever tried substance | Percent of parents who reported last month drug use |
|---|---|---|
| cigarettes | 43.5 | 28.3 |
| alcohol | 56.6 | 26.1 |
| marijuana | 10.9 | 2.2 |
| inhalants | 0.0 | 0.0 |
| cocaine | 2.2 | 0.0 |
| other drugs | 2.2 | 2.2 |

## *Identification of Other Drug Users*

Responses to six questions assessed the parents' perceptions of their friends and families ATOD use (N = 49). Table 2 depicts the actual percentages of affirmative responses on each question. Parents reported high percentages of their friends and family used alcohol, 73.3% and 71.7% respectively. As far as marijuana use, parents reported that 13.3% of their friends and 17.4% of their family used this substance. In addition, parents reported that 4.3% of their friends used other drugs.

Approximately 20 parents and 68 youth participated in the family camps for a total of 88 unduplicated participants. The average attendance for each family camp was 13 persons. An average of 9 parents attended each family support group., A core group of 18 parents became regular participants at these family support groups. An average parent attended slightly over three support groups with a total of 14.6 hours attended by each parent.

*Test of hypothesis one.* Mean scores, for both the pretest and the posttests, were compiled for each of the sub-scales of FACES III. The results of independent sample t-tests, using an alpha level of .05 for a one tail test, indicated no differences in pretest and posttest mean scores for *Cohesion* (see Table 3), *Adaptability* (see Table 4), and *Family type* (see Table 5).

TABLE 2. Percent of Parents Reporting They Have Friends and Family Who Use Alcohol or Drugs (N = 49)

| Substance | Percentage |
|---|---|
| Alcohol use by friends | 73.3 |
| Marijuana use by friends | 13.3 |
| Other drug use by friends | 4.3 |
| Marijuana use by family | 17.4 |
| Alcohol use by family | 71.7 |
| Other drug use by family | N/A |

### Test of Hypothesis Two

For the drug knowledge questionnaire, the average percentage of correct responses at pretest and posttest was calculated for each question, and then the percent of change was calculated (see Table 6). Comparing pretest and posttest, the percentage of correct responses increased on 16 out of 20 questions. The overall average percentage of correct responses was 58.8 (N = 49) on the pretest and 68.2 (N = 32) on the posttest. This reflected a 9.4 average point improvement of scores.

## DISCUSSION

The parents had a mean score of 1.9 giving them a strong Mexican orientation. This finding was consistent with our expectation that the first generation holds to their culture of origin. This finding is significant because it indicated that we had a group of "Mexican thinking" parents whose concept of drug use did not really include drug abuse. In other words, the parents did not have concepts for drug abuse, and thus, were not really equipped to deal with their children's drug abuse issues. This fact of lack of awareness, or lack of knowledge of the concepts of abuse, not only indicated a high risk population, but the necessity to vary the intervention according to the acculturation level. This study attempted to do just that, adjusting the intervention to the acculturation level of the parents. Basic features of the program included the staff being bi-lingual, and all parent questionnaires were available in Spanish as well as English.

TABLE 3. Cohesion Scores for Parents Before and After Intervention Programs (N = 32)

| Pretest | Posttest | Difference |
|---|---|---|
| 3.75 | 4.16 | −.41 |
| $t = -.81$, $df = 31$, $p = .21$ | | |

The cohesion scores are categorized as follows:
1 and 2 = *disengaged*; 3 and 4 = *separated*;
5 and 6 = *connected*; 7 and 8 = *very connected.*

TABLE 4. Adaptability Scores for Parents Before and After Intervention Programs (N = 32)

| Pretest | Posttest | Difference |
|---|---|---|
| 5.1 | 4.5 | 0.6 |
| $t = 1.09$, $df = 31$, $p = .42$ | | |

The adaptability scores are categorized as follows:
1 and 2 = *rigid*; 3 and 4 = *structured*;
5 and 6 = *flexible*; 7 and 8 = *very flexible*.

TABLE 5. Family Type Scores for Parents Before and After Intervention Programs (N = 32)

| Pretest | Posttest | Difference |
|---|---|---|
| 4.44 | 4.36 | .08 |
| $t = .18$, $df = 31$, $p = .43$ | | |

The family type scores are categorized as follows:
1 and 2 = *extreme*; 3 and 4 = *mid-range*;
5 and 6 = *moderately balanced*; 7 and 8 = *balanced*.

Although a research hypothesis concerning parent drug use was not included in the study, the findings were noteworthy. Parent drug use appeared to be somewhat low; this may be due to the all female sample that might tend to have lower usage levels than a male or a mixed group. Despite assurance of confidentiality, the factor of "social desirability" may have resulted in participants reporting lower use than the actual facts. Nonetheless, since a relationship between parents' and children's drug use has been reported in the literature, the current findings about the drug usage of parents serves to alert professionals to the potential risk for children's drug use.

There was no evidence to support the hypothesis that the FACES III scores on cohesiveness, adaptability, or family type improved from pretest to posttest. It can be said that overall, the parents were functioning in the mid-range category. The mid-range category is the approximate

TABLE 6. Percent of Correct Responses on Pretest and Posttest, and Pretest to Posttest Change, for Parents' Responses to Drug Knowledge Questions

| # | Drug Knowledge Question | Percentage correct on pretest (N = 49) | Percentage correct on posttest (N = 32) | Pretest to posttest change* |
|---|---|---|---|---|
| 1 | Frequent drinkers need alcohol to feel good. | 66.0 | 63.6 | −2.4 |
| 2 | Pot helps people remember things. | 67.4 | 72.7 | 5.3 |
| 3 | The effects of pot on growing persons is unknown. | 29.5 | 27.3 | −2.2 |
| 4 | Frequent use of inhalants may cause brain damage. | 93.6 | 100.0 | 6.4 |
| 5 | Barbiturate users can stop without side effects. | 58.7 | 61.3 | 2.6 |
| 6 | When the effects of cocaine are over, the user feels happy. | 52.2 | 60.6 | 8.4 |
| 7 | Pot may make the user feel afraid. | 28.9 | 30.3 | 1.4 |
| 8 | Cocaine does not harm the body of the user. | 70.2 | 78.8 | 8.6 |
| 9 | Smoking crack is safer than sniffing cocaine. | 63.8 | 76.2 | 12.4 |
| 10 | Anxiety reaction refers to the anxiety sensation from smoking pot. | 36.2 | 50.0 | 13.8 |
| 11 | Smoking crack will not produce symptoms of cocaine use. | 36.2 | 57.6 | 21.4 |
| 12 | Alcohol related car accidents are the number one cause of teenage deaths. | 83.0 | 93.9 | 10.9 |
| 13 | Regular cocaine use rarely causes addiction. | 46.8 | 78.8 | 3.2 |
| 14 | Smoking cigarettes is harmful to the unborn child. | 97.8 | 97.0 | −0.8 |
| 15 | Regular use of uppers may cause harm. | 87.2 | 87.5 | 0.3 |
| 16 | Smoking pot improves driving ability. | 74.2 | 72.7 | 1.8 |
| 17 | It is easy to overdose on barbiturates when mixing with alcohol. | 70.2 | 78.8 | 8.6 |
| 18 | Cocaine may produce symptoms of paranoia. | 55.3 | 63.6 | 8.3 |
| 19 | Pot smoke is less cancer causing than cigarette smoke. | 26.1 | 21.9 | −4.2 |
| 20 | Sharing drug needles increases the risk of contracting AIDS. | 32.7 | 90.9 | 58.2 |

*Negative numbers indicated that percentage of correct responses went down at posttest, while positive numbers indicated that percentage of correct responses increased.

mid-point between the two extremes on the continuum of family types, and is typical of a desirable score range for a family.

There were a few factors that could account for the lack of differences from pretest to posttest on FACES III scores. Due to self-selection of the sample, perhaps only relatively well functioning families entered into the study. Also, since pretest scores of these participants were in a desirable range, a major change in posttest scores was not likely for the group. A future study with families known to have less than desirable functioning might better test whether the intervention used affected family functioning. Another related explanation of lack of change is that the intervention may not have been long enough in duration to effect a change in family functioning. Additionally, the statistical test used may not have been adequate in detecting a difference. It would have been preferable to match parents on their pretest and posttest scores. Paired difference scores of individual parents were unavailable for analysis due to lack of a coding system in the data collection phase. Had scores been matched for a stronger analysis, and still pre-post comparisons failed to reveal significant differences, individual family change could have been investigated as a possible avenue to more effectively apply future interventions. A final reason that a change did not emerge from the analysis could be that the instruments, translated from English to Spanish, simply were not meaningful to the respondents or did not measure what they intended to measure. Concepts of family functioning translated to Spanish may lose the original meaning by which they were developed and tested in English. The FACES III has been used previously in Spanish and Puerto Rican populations in the eastern United States and Mexican American populations in Los Angeles (J. J. Paz, personal communication, February 9, 2004). Data on utilization of the translated FACES III, as well as information on its discriminate validity, would support assessment of its validity with Latino populations.

The Census Bureau Office of Management and Budget defined Hispanic or Latino as "a person of Cuban, Mexican, Puerto Rican, South or Central American, or other Spanish culture or origin regardless of race" (Grieco & Cassidy, 2001). While most participants in the current study identified themselves as Mexican Americans (79%), families from Cuba or South America who are newly arriving in the United States and/or are not yet highly acculturated may have similarities to the study sample.

The data revealed preliminary evidence that a culturally competent approach improved drug knowledge of Latino parents. While the 9.4

average improvement of scores was indicative of a positive trend, this evidence needs to be considered with caution. As in English, Spanish drug terminology varies with locality, and by county/culture of origin. There may be concepts imbedded in the English instrument that when translated to the Spanish version, do not accurately reflect what the instrument was intended to measure.

However, if drug knowledge of parents can improve by any degree, there is potential for parents to influence and improve their children's drug knowledge and awareness. This potential for influence may be an important key for prevention of drug abuse. The *Proyecto Juventud* project is currently being replicated with urban Latino adolescents in Tucson, Arizona. The program known as *Corazon de Aztlan* (funded by the Center for Substance Abuse Prevention) is under the auspices of *Chicanos Por La Causa* and has attained similar outcomes (J. J. Paz, personal communication, February 9, 2004). Model program descriptions and outcomes are available as resources for social workers interested in learning about and/or implementing a prevention program with Latino families and youth at risk for substance abuse and other related high-risk behaviors (Substance Abuse and Mental Health Services Administration National Registry of Effective Programs, 2002). As Chavez (1999) noted, parents are vital sources of guidance in the Latino community, and it is imperative that parents use their influence to counteract the likelihood that their children will engage in substance abuse. This study illustrates the importance of addressing cultural issues as social workers attempt to effect change in the Latino family.

## REFERENCES

Acosta, A., & Hamel, V. (1995). *Hispanic/Latino natural support systems: Center for Substance Abuse Prevention implementation guide* (Monograph, DHHS-SMA-95-3033). Washington, DC: U.S. Government Printing Office.

Austin, G. A., & Pollard, J. A. (1993). *Substance abuse and ethnicity: Recent research findings* (Prevention research update 10). Portland, OR: Western Regional Center Drug-Free Schools and Communities Northwest Regional Educational Laboratory.

Barrera Jr., M., & Li, S. A. (1993). Ethnic group differences in vulnerability to parental alcoholism and life stress: A study of Hispanic and non-Hispanic Caucasian adolescents. *American Journal of Community Psychology, 21*(1), 15-35.

Barrera Jr., M., & Li, S. A. (1995). Effects of parental alcoholism and life stress on Hispanic. *American Journal of Community Psychology, 23*(4), 479.

Barrera Jr., M., Li, S. A., & Chassin, L. (1998). Exploring adolescents' vulnerability to life stress and parental alcoholism: The role of ethnicity and family conflict. In H. I.

McCubbin, & E. A. Thompson et al. (Eds.), *Resiliency in Native American and immigrant families* (pp. 295-324). Thousand Oaks, CA: Sage Publications, Inc.

Chavez, N. (1999). *Hablemos en confienza, Hispanic/Latino initiative is launched to reduce substance abuse*. Substance Abuse and Mental Health Services Administration. Retrieved March 12, 2001, from the World Wide Web: *www.samhsa.gov/press/99/991004nr.htm*

Coombs, R. H., Paulson, M. J., & Richardson, M. A. (1991). Peer vs. parental influence in substance abuse among Hispanic and Anglo children and adolescents. *Journal of Youth & Adolescence, 20*(1), 73-88.

Cuellar, I., Arnold, B., & Maldonado, R. (1995). Acculturation rating scale for Mexican Americans-II: A revision of the original ARSMA scale. *Hispanic Journal of Behavioral Sciences, 17*(2), 275-301.

Delgado, M. (1995). Hispanic natural support systems and alcohol and other drug services: Challenges and rewards for practice. *Alcoholism Treatment Quarterly, 12*(1), 17-31.

Delgado, M. (1996). Implementing a natural support system AOD project: Administrative considerations and recommendations. *Alcoholism Treatment Quarterly, 14*(2), 1-14.

Delgado, M. (1998a). Cultural competence and the field of ATOD: Latinos as a case example. *Alcoholism Treatment Quarterly, 16*(1-2).

Delgado, M. (1998b). *Social services in Latino communities: Research and strategies*. New York: The Haworth Press, Inc.

Department of Health and Human Services. (1995). *A Hispanic/Latino family approach to substance abuse prevention: Center for Substance Abuse Prevention cultural competence series 2* (Monograph, DHHS-SMA-95-3034). Washington, DC: U.S. Government Printing Office.

Figueroa-Moseley, C. D. V. (1998). Latino youth substance use and abuse: Some findings from the Hispanic health and nutrition examination survey. *Dissertation Abstracts International: Section B: The Sciences & Engineering, 58*(12-B), 6518.

Fischer, J., & Corcoran, K. (1994). *Measures for clinical practice: A sourcebook* (2nd ed.). New York: Free Press.

Flores, M. T., & Carey, G. (2000). *Family therapy with Hispanics: Toward appreciating diversity*. Boston: Allyn and Bacon.

Geroerer, J., & De La Rosa, M. R. (1993). Protective and risk factors associated with drug use among Hispanic youth. *Journal of Addictive Diseases, 12*(2), 87-107.

Gilbert, M. J., Solis, B., & Mora, J. (1992). *Alcohol-related issues in the Latino population, 1980-1990: An annotated bibliography*. Berkeley: Chicano Studies Library Publication Unit University of California at Berkeley.

Glick, R., & Moore, J. W. (1990). *Drugs in Hispanic communities*. New Brunswick: Rutgers University Press.

Grieco, E. M., & Cassidy, R. C. (2001). *Overview of race and Hispanic origin: Census 2000 brief*. Retrieved February 8, 2004, from the World Wide Web: http://*www.census.gov/prod/2001pubs/c2kbr01-1.pdf*

Hawkins, J. D., Catalano, R. F., & Miller, J. Y. (1992). Risk and protective factors for alcohol and other drug problems in adolescence and early adulthood: Implications for substance abuse prevention. *Psychological Bulletin, 112*, 64-105.

Hernandez, L. P., & Lucero, E. (1996). Denver area youth services la familia community drug and alcohol prevention program: Family-centered model for working with inner-city Hispanic families. *The Journal of Primary Prevention, 16*(3), 255-272.

Johnson, J. L., & Leff, M. (1999). Children of substance abusers: Overview of research findings. *Pediatrics, 103*(5), 1085-1099.

Johnson, P. B., & Johnson, H. L. (1999). Cultural and family influences that maintain the negative meaning of alcohol. *Journal of Studies on Alcohol, 60*(2), 79.

Kar, S. B. (1999). *Substance abuse prevention: A multicultural perspective*. Amityville, NY: Baywood.

Krestan, J. A. (2000). *Bridges to recovery: Addiction, family therapy, and multicultural treatment*. New York: Free Press.

Krohn, M. D., & Thornberry, T. P. (1993). Network theory: A model for understanding drug abuse among African American and Hispanic youth. *National Institute on Drug Abuse Research Monograph Series, 130*, 102-128.

Lewis, M. D., Beavers, W. R., Gosset, J. T., & Phillips, V. A. (1976). *No single thread: Psychological health in family systems*. New York: Brunner/Mazel.

Maddahian, E., Newcomb, M. D., & Bentler, P. M. (1988). Risk factors for substance use: Ethnic differences among adolescents. *Journal of Substance Abuse, 1*(1), 11-23.

Mayers, R. S., Kail, B. L., & Watts, T. D. (Eds.). (1993). *Hispanic substance abuse*. Springfield: Charles C Thomas.

McClanahan, T. M. (1998). *A concise and practical guide to family assessment*. Paper presented at the Annual Conference of American Psychological Association, San Francisco, CA.

Olsen, D. H. (1986). Circumplex Model VII: Validation studies and FACES-III. *Family Process, 25*, 337-351.

Perez, W., & Padilla, A. M. (2000). Cultural orientation across three generations of Hispanic adolescents. *Hispanic Journal of Behavioral Sciences, 22*(3), 30-39.

Rhodes, J. E., & Jason, L. A. (1990). A social stress model of substance abuse. *Journal of Consulting & Clinical Psychology, 58*(4), 395-401.

Santisteban, D. A., Szapocznik, J., & Rio, A. T. (1993). Family therapy for Hispanic substance abusing youth. In R. S. Mayers, & B. L. Kail et al. (Eds.), *Hispanic substance abuse* (pp. 157-173). Springfield: Charles C Thomas.

Scheier, L. M., Botvin, G. J., & Miller, N. L. (1999). Life events, neighborhood stress, psychosocial functioning, and alcohol use among urban minority youth. *Journal of Child & Adolescent Substance Abuse, 9*(1), 19-50.

Sealy, Y. M. (2000). The relationship between parenting behaviors and alcohol consumption of Hispanic and African males during adolescence and young adulthood. *Dissertation Abstracts International, 60*(9), 3529A. (UMI No. DA9947099).

Sokol-Katz, J. S., & Ulbrich, P. M. (1992). Family structure and adolescent risk-taking behavior: A comparison of Mexican, Cuban, and Puerto Rican Americans. *International Journal of the Addictions, 27*(10), 1197-1209.

Sotomayor, M. (1991). *Empowering Hispanic families: A critical issue for the '90s*. Milwaukee, WI: Family Service America.

Substance Abuse and Mental Health Services Administration National Registry of Effective Programs. (2002). *Effective substance abuse and mental health programs for every community*. Retrieved February 9, 2004, from the World Wide Web: *http://modelprograms.samhsa.gov/template.cfm?page=default*

Szapocznik, J., Amaro, H., & U.S. Dept. of Health and Human Services. (1995). *A Hispanic/Latino family approach to substance abuse prevention: Center for Substance Abuse Prevention cultural competence series 2* (xiv, 207 p.). Washington, DC: U.S. Government Printing Office.

Szapocznik, J., Perez-Vidal, A., Brickman, A. L., Foote, F. H., Santisteban, D. A., Hervis, O., & Kurtines, W. M. (1989). Engaging adolescent drug abusers and their families in treatment: A strategic-structural systems approach. *Journal of Consulting & Clinical Psychology, 56*(4), 552-557.

Vega, W. A., & Gil, A. G. (1998). *Drug use and ethnicity in early adolescence*. New York: Plenum Press.

Vega, W. A., Kourney, E. I., Zimmerman, R. S., & Gil, A. G. (1995). Cultural conflicts and problem behaviors of Latino adolescents in home and school environments. *Journal of Community Psychology, 23*, 167-179.

Wallace, J. M. (1999). The social ecology of addiction: Race, risk, and resilience. *Pediatrics, 103*(5), 1122-1127.

# Psychiatric, Family, and Ethnicity-Related Factors That Can Impact Treatment Utilization Among Hispanic Substance Abusing Adolescents

Daniel A. Santisteban
Frank Dillon
Maite P. Mena
Yannine Estrada
Ellen L. Vaughan

Daniel A. Santisteban, PhD, Frank Dillon, PhD, Maite P. Mena, PsyD, Yannine Estrada, BA, and Ellen L. Vaughan, MA, are affiliated with the Center for Family Studies, Department of Psychiatry and Behavioral Sciences, University of Miami.

Address correspondence to: Daniel A. Santisteban, PhD, Miller School of Medicine, University of Miami, Center for Family Studies, 1425 Northwest 10th Avenue, 3rd Floor, Miami, FL 33136 (E-mail: dsantist@med.miami.edu).

The authors would like to thank the Juvenile Addiction Receiving Facility Unit Director Eve Sakran, and Medical Directors, Drs. Hector Biaggi and Louis Antoine. They would like to acknowledge the contributions of JARF Director, Eve Sakran, Medical Director, Hector Biaggi, and the entire staff of the unit for their dedication to improving the lives of their clients.

This work was funded by (National Institute on Drug Abuse) Grant No. 1 RO1 DA 13104, Developing a Culturally-Rooted Adolescent Family Therapy–Daniel A. Santisteban, PhD, Principal Investigator, and Grant No. 1U1ODA 13720. Florida Node of the Drug Abuse Clinical Trials Network–José Szapocznik, PhD, Principal Investigator.

[Haworth co-indexing entry note]: "Psychiatric, Family, and Ethnicity-Related Factors That Can Impact Treatment Utilization Among Hispanic Substance Abusing Adolescents." Santisteban, Daniel A. et al. Co-published simultaneously in *Journal of Social Work Practice in the Addictions* (The Haworth Press, Inc.) Vol. 5, No. 1/2, 2005, pp. 133-155; and: *Substance Abusing Latinos: Current Research on Epidemiology, Prevention, and Treatment* (ed: Mario R. De La Rosa, Lori K. Holleran, and Shulamith Lala Ashenberg Straussner) The Haworth Press, Inc., 2005, pp. 133-155. Single or multiple copies of this article are available for a fee from The Haworth Document Delivery Service [1-800-HAWORTH, 9:00 a.m. - 5:00 p.m. (EST). E-mail address: docdelivery@haworthpress.com].

http://www.haworthpress.com/web/JSWPA

Digital Object Identifier: 10.1300/J160v05n01_07

**SUMMARY.** There is great significance to improving our understanding of predictors of treatment utilization among Hispanic substance abusing youth. One hundred and ten Hispanic substance abusing adolescents and their parents participated in a study of treatment utilization. Analyses showed that adolescents with lower numbers of externalizing disorders ($\chi^2 = 4.18$, $df = 1$, $p < .05$) and parents with better parenting strategies ($\chi^2 = 8.73$, $df = 2$, $p < .05$), predicted overall treatment utilization (residential + outpatient). Better parenting practices and higher parental years in the U.S. predicted more utilization of outpatient services and lower parenting stress predicted more utilization of residential services. Without specialized engagement strategies, adolescents and families most in need may be the least likely to engage in recommended treatment. 

**KEYWORDS.** Hispanic adolescents, treatment utilization, substance abuse, parenting strategies

## *INTRODUCTION*

It is widely accepted that a small minority of youth requiring treatment for a diagnosable disorder actually ever receive treatment (The National Advisory Mental Health Council Workgroup on Child and Adolescent Mental Health Intervention Development and Deployment, 2001) and this is particularly true among substance abusing youth (Szapocznik et al., 1988). In 2002, approximately 1.4 million youths between the age of 12 to 17 required treatment for a drug abuse problem. Of these, only ten percent (approximately 140,000) received treatment, with the remaining 90% of youths who needed substance use treatment failing to receive it (Substance Abuse and Mental Health Service Administration (SAMHSA), 2002. This low level of treatment utilization among adolescents has important implications not only for the alleviation of their current symptomatology but also for the progression of these problems into more serious forms of psychopathology in adulthood (Logan & King, 2001).

The underutilization of treatment appears to be even more severe among Hispanics. In a review of mental health services for Hispanics (not specific to adolescents), Rogler (1998) notes that despite high rates of affective disorders and co-morbidity, there is still significant underutilization of mental health services by Hispanics. Recent studies examining service utilization among minority adolescents have found that Hispanic adolescents use mental health services at rates lower than their non-Hispanic white counterparts (Goodman et al., 1997; Hough et al., 2002; Wu, Hoven, & Fuller, 2003). Results from the Methodology for the Epidemiology of Child and Adolescent Mental Disorders (MECA) study found that the percentage of non-Hispanic white adolescents using outpatient mental health services was approximately twice the rate of minorities in the sample (Goodman et al., 1997). In addition to finding lower outpatient utilization for Latino youth, Hough and colleagues (2002) found that Latinos were older when they began attending services. Interestingly, the finding by Wu, Hoven, and Fuller (2003) that minority youth had lower rates of utilization of drug treatment was diminished after controlling for drug use severity and other related problems. These authors suggest that lower minority utilization of services may have been partly explained by their lower drug use rates.

There is great clinical significance to the field of social work and other related fields, to better understanding the types of psychiatric, family, and ethnicity-related factors that can impact service utilization and specifically, follow-up on recommended substance abuse treatment services. The impact of programs that conduct assessments and referral of youth with psychiatric problems is greatly diminished when youth and families do not engage into the recommended treatment. An improved understanding of the predictors of failure to engage in treatment can lead to more specialized and targeted interventions that will increase the probability of engagement. Consequently, the purpose of this article is to report on the findings of a study that (1) focused on Hispanic drug abusing adolescents and their families, (2) systematically assessed a number of important psychiatric, family, and ethnicity-related characteristics, and (3) investigated the relationship of these important variables to later engagement into recommended substance abuse services.

## *PREDICTORS OF UTILIZATION OF RECOMMENDED SERVICES*

### *Adolescent Psychopathology*

Two of the factors consistently related to service utilization are problem severity and co-morbidity (Goodman et al., 1997; Pumariega,

Glover, Holzer, & Nguyen, 1998; Wu et al., 2003; Wu, Hoven, Tiet, Kovalenko, & Wicks, 2002). Goodman and colleagues (1997) examined data from the MECA study and found that those adolescents with any disorder who attended outpatient mental health services had significantly lower mean scores on a global assessment measure and were more likely to have co-morbid disorders than those with any disorder who did not attend mental health services. Overall, this study indicates that those attending services had *more impairment in functioning*. Similarly, in a study using a sample of junior and high school students, Pumariega and colleagues (1998) found that the total Youth Self-Report (YSR) score was predictive of service utilization with an increase in use of mental health services as symptomatology increased. Interestingly, this result emerged using the total sample (488 non-white Hispanics, 194 Hispanics, and 102 African-Americans), but did not emerge within the Hispanic subsample. Wu et al. (2003) also examined severity and co-morbidity as predictors of drug treatment among adolescents reporting drug use in the past year, finding that more severe drug-related problems and multiple drug use predicted utilization of drug treatment. Overall, the findings from these studies suggest that among adolescents greater service utilization is related to more severe symptomatology and co-occurring disorders.

### *Socio-Demographic Variables*

Family composition and economic variables have been found to be associated with service utilization. Economic obstacles can take many forms in their impact on whether or not substance-specific services are utilized by Hispanic youth. Some youth may not have the availability of needed services (Johnson, Stiffman, Hadley-Ives, & Elze, 2001). Even when these services are available, additional economic obstacles can hinder service utilization by Hispanic adolescents (Pumariega et al., 1998). The direct effects of poverty, such as not being able to afford transportation, parents not being able to take time off from work to accompany adolescents through the process, and other limited resources are powerful enough to undermine service use, even in the presence of government funded agencies designed to provide services for low income groups. Family composition has also been suggested as a factor associated with Hispanic adolescent's receipt of mental health services. Families with a large number of siblings are often less likely to use mental health services and females appeared more likely than males to receive services (Pumariega et al., 1998).

### *Family and Parental Predictors*

Another set of important predictors of adolescent service utilization are family factors and parent functioning, although the precise nature of the relationship remains very unclear (Cornelius, Pringle, Jernigan, Kirisci, & Clark, 2001; Farmer, Burns, Angold, & Costello, 1997). Parental well-being and parental feelings of competence in dealing with their children's problem have been negatively associated with service use as the parents of high utilization youth reported lower levels of both well-being and feelings of competence (Farmer et al., 1997). The presence of family stress (in this study due to changes in family composition) has been associated with increased service utilization (Zwaanswijk, Van der Ende, Verhaak, Bensing, & Verhulst, 2003).

Logan and King (2001) present a converging literature on service utilization by both adults and child/adolescents suggesting that family history of psychological problems may increase the likelihood of service use. However, research examining mental health service use among male adolescents suggests that parental psychopathology and parental substance abuse can act as deterrents to adequate mental health treatment by adolescents (Cornelius et al., 2001). These apparently inconsistent findings on the effects of parental psychopathology may depend on the overall level of psychopathology of the parent. It is worth considering whether some history of problems may lead to a heightened awareness of the need for services when compared to parents with no history of problems, but severe problems may lead to obstacles to utilization.

### *Ethnicity-Related Factors*

The evaluation of ethnicity-related factors associated with service use among Hispanics is important given that the lack of culturally specific services is often cited as a major factor in service underutilization by Hispanics (Rogler, 1998). A study by Takeuchi, Sue, and Yeh (1998) found that Mexican-American adult clients attending ethnicity specific programs had higher return rates and longer lengths of treatment. Little is known, however, about cultural factors, including acculturation, as predictors of service utilization in adolescents (Hough et al., 2002; Pumariega et al., 1998). Pumariega and colleagues (1998) collected data on items typically associated with acculturation (e.g., place of birth, self-rating of English fluency, and self-rated reading and writing in English) and found that immigrant youth and youth who rated themselves as speaking English poorly had more mental health visits than those born in the U.S. and those rating themselves as speaking English well. Interestingly, the same relationship was not found for ability to read and write English. In addition, it is also important to disentangle the role of ethnicity from the role that socioeconomic status plays in service utilization (Pumariega et al., 1998). Although Logan and King found an overall pattern of higher service utilization by Caucasian and urban families with strong economic circumstances, Pumariega and colleagues (1998) found that when socioeconomic factors are controlled for, there were no differences in service utilization by Hispanics and African Americans when compared to whites.

## *METHOD*

### *Participants*

Participants in this study were 110 Hispanic adolescents and their parents. Adolescents had been admitted to an assessment and referral facility, Juvenile Addiction Receiving Facility at Jackson Hospital, due to substance use problems. The mean age of the adolescents was 15.6 years (SD = 1.96) and the median age was 16-years-old. Sixty percent of the sample was male. Mother reports were much more common than father reports and are therefore the focus of analyses. Mother's reported ethnicities were: 40% Cuban, 12% Honduran, 9% Puerto Rican, 8% Dominican, 8% Nicaraguan, 7% Columbian, and 16% other Hispanic. Sixty-six percent of the youth were U.S. born while 34% where born in Hispanic countries. Eighty-one percent of mothers reported an educational level of high school or less. Sixty-one percent of the families reported an annual household income of $25,000 or less, 12% between $25,000 and $29,999, and 27% above $30,000. The median family income range for the sample was between $20,000 and $24,999.

To be included in the study, the adolescent/families had to meet the following criteria: (a) Hispanic adolescent 14- to 17-years-old; (b) adolescent living with at least one family member of an older generation such as a parent or grandparent, also Hispanic and having immigrated to the U.S.; and (c) adolescent fully meeting Diagnostic and Statistical Manual IV (DSM IV) criteria for a Substance Abuse or Dependency Disorder. Adolescents with signs of the following DSM-IV diagnoses were not included in the study: Developmental Disorders, Elective Mutism, Organic Mental Disorders (except Psychoactive Substance-Induced), Schizophrenia, Delusional (Paranoid) Disorder, Psychotic Disorder, and Bipolar Affective Disorder.

### *Procedure*

All participant adolescents were recruited from the Juvenile Addictions Receiving Facility (JARF) of a local southeastern hospital where adolescents had been admitted for assessment of their substance abuse problem and were referred to treatment in the community. The records of new admissions to the JARF were screened at least twice per week by a trained bachelor's level, Spanish-speaking research assistant to determine eligibility. Once an adolescent was determined to be eligible for the research program, a social worker on the unit obtained permission from the primary caregiver and the adolescent for the research assistant to contact them in order to explain the research program. The research assistant, then, contacted those potential participants who had given permission and explained to them the research program, that participation would require both parents and the adolescent to complete a one-time assessment which would take approximately 3 hours and that they would receive $40 for their participation. Additionally, all participants were told that they would be contacted via telephone six weeks after the adolescent had been discharged to complete a 10-minute questionnaire about follow-up services received by the adolescent since being discharged. Both adolescents and parents were informed that their information would be kept confidential. Seventy-four percent of the families approached agreed to participate in the research. Upon signing the consent and assent forms, parents and adolescents were administered the assessment battery consisting of both self-report measures and semi-structured interviews.

### *Measures*

For this study, measures were selected that addressed substance use, parenting practices, stress, attachment, psychiatric comorbidity, acculturation, demographic information, and the utilization of treatment services following discharge. Adolescents were administered the battery while they were on the JARF unit and parents were administered the battery at the research office or in their home. Spanish language measures were available to those adolescents and parents who were more comfortable speaking and reading in Spanish. Parents and children were asked if they would like the questionnaire read to them, in the event that they had difficulty reading. The interview to assess service utilization was done over the phone using a semi-structured interview.

*Substance use*. The Personal Experiences Inventory (PEI) is a standardized inventory used to provide descriptive information concerning adolescent drug use and problems associated with drug use (Winters & Henly, 1989). It is organized into a Chemical Involvement Problem Severity Section and a Psychosocial Section that comprise a total of 22 subscales. Additionally, there is a drug use frequency, duration, and age of onset section. Questions in the section inquire about frequency of drug use for twelve drug categories over the past 12 months and 3 months and lifetime use. Additional questions ask the school grade in which the respondent began using each of the drugs. Its overall psychometric properties have been found to be satisfactory with internal consistency coefficient alphas ranging from .74 to .97 for all 22 scales. The PEI has also been shown to have satisfactory test-retest reliability with coefficients ranging from .63 to .90 on all scales using a one-month interval with a wait list clinical sample. The drug use frequency, duration, and age of onset section was the only section used in the analyses reported in this manuscript.

*Parenting practices.* The Parenting Practices Questionnaire (Gorman-Smith, Tolan, Zelli, & Huesmann, 1996; Loeber, Stouthamer-Loeber; Van Kammen & Farrington, 1991) assesses five dimensions of parenting behavior: positive parenting, discipline effectiveness, discipline avoidance, rules on having a set time to be home, and extent of involvement. Parents are asked to report on all five dimensions while adolescent reports are obtained for positive parenting and extent of involvement only. The reliability of the scales has been supported by confirmatory factor analysis and internal consistency has been measured as ranging from .68 to .81 in past studies. Alphas ranged from .73 to .89 in the current study.

*Stress.* The Hispanic Stress Inventory (HSI) (Cervantes, Padilla, Salgado de Snyder, 1991) is a culturally sensitive self-report questionnaire designed to measure psychosocial stress levels among Hispanic respondents (Cervantes et al., 1991). The HSI has two versions, one for Hispanic immigrant respondents and one for U.S. born Hispanic respondents. Each version has a subscale for occupational/economic stress, parenting stress, marital stress, and family/culture stress. The immigrant version has an additional subscale for immigration stress and was the version used in our study. Respondents are first asked whether they have experienced a stressor, encompassed within one of the subscales, in the last three months. If the respondent answers "yes," they received a score of one for each item. If they respond "no" to the occurrence of the stressor, they received a score of zero. Subscale scores were obtained by summing respective items. Following the recommendation of the measure's author, the adolescents completed only the family/culture subscale thus they received a shortened 13-item version of the HIS while the parents received the full version. Indicators of internal consistency were high for the Immigrant version, ranging from .91 for Occupational/Economic Stress to .77 for Family/Cultural Stress. Test-retest reliability for the Immigrant version ranged from .86 for Family/Cultural Stress to .61 for Marital Stress. Alphas for the current sample range from .73 to .85.

*Attachment.* The Inventory of Parent and Peer Attachment (IPPA) (Armsden & Greenberg, 1987) was developed to assess adolescent perception of the positive and negative aspects of their attachment to their parents. In this study we focused only on adolescent reports of adolescent-mother attachment. The IPPA is a self-report measure of three dimensions: degree of mutual trust, quality of communication, and the extent of anger and alienation. Internal consistency, measured by Cronbach's alpha, was .87 for the mother version and .89 for the father version. Alphas for the current sample ranged from .75 to .88. The IPPA was shown to have a correlation coefficient of .78 with family self-concept as assessed by the Tennessee Self-Concept Scale and .52 with family expressiveness on the Family Environment Scale (Armsden & Greenberg, 1987). The IPPA was administered as a self-report to the adolescents.

*Psychiatric comorbidity.* The Diagnostic Interview Schedule for Children-Predictive Scales (DPS version 4.21) was administered separately to parents and adolescents in interview format. This measure is an efficient screening instrument made up of a series of diagnostic scales matched to the Diagnostic Interview Schedule for Children (DISC). It evaluates the likelihood that a child does not meet diagnostic criteria for a psychiatric diagnosis and those that should be further evaluated with the DISC (Lucas et al., 2001). Scores are obtained for each psychiatric disorder and the presence of symptoms of a diagnosis is based on cut-offs for psychiatric disorders established in previous research with clinical samples. Internal consistency for the DPS as measured by coefficient alphas was Attention Deficit Hyperactivity Disorder–0.82; Depression–0.77; Oppositional Defiant Disorder–0.75; Conduct Disorder–0.69 (Lucas et al., 2001). Using the DPS as a self-report questionnaire followed by the full DISC, Lucas et al. (2001) found that from a total of 75 diagnoses only 3 diagnoses were missed by gate items from the DPS (n = 89). Sensitivity with respect to the DISC for specific DPS scales was Attention Deficit Hyperactivity Disorder–1.00; Depression–0.98; Oppositional Defiant Disorder–0.96; Conduct Disorder–1.00 and for specificity, Attention Deficit Hyperactivity Disorder– 0.85; Depression–0.90; Oppositional Defiant Disorder–0.94; Conduct Disorder-0.94 (Lucas et al., 2001).

*Acculturation.* The Bicultural Involvement Questionnaire (Szapocznik, Kurtines, & Fernandez, 1980) is a 33-item questionnaire designed to assess the degree to which an individual participates and feels comfortable in Hispanic culture and activities (Hispanicism score) and in American culture and activities (Americanism score) independently. The measure differs from those that are unidimensional (e.g., Szapocznik, Scopetta, Kurtines, & Arnalde, 1978) which assume that participation and comfort in one culture negates the possibility of participation and comfort in another. The Bicultural Involvement Questionnaire is rated on a 5-point Likert scale. Aggregate scores for two dimensions of bicultural involvement can be obtained. The first dimension ranges from monoculturalism to biculturalism. The second dimension is cultural involvement, and ranges from culturally marginal (lacks involvement in either the Hispanic or the American culture) to cultural involvement. Previous research has found alpha internal consistency coefficients of .93 and .89 for Hispanicism and Americanism scales, respectively. The Biculturalism and Cultural Involvement scales were found to have reliability coefficients of .94 and .79, respectively (Szapocznik et al., 1980).

*Demographics.* An intake form was created specifically for this study to collect demographic information, including the family's ethnicity, religious preference, family composition, biological parents' marital living status, household income, age of onset for drug (non-alcohol) use, and language preference. Also included in this form were questions about prior adolescent residential/inpatient treatment for drug use and/ or outpatient treatment for drug use, and adolescent/parent separations lasting longer than one month and not due to vacationing.

*Follow-up questionnaire.* The follow-up questionnaire consisted of a semi-structured interview designed specifically for the current study. The primary caregiver of the participant adolescent was contacted via telephone 6 weeks after the adolescent was discharged and was administered the follow-up questionnaire to document utilization of services by the adolescent post-discharge. Questions ask whether or not the adolescent was referred for treatment upon discharge from the JARF, which type of treatment they were referred to (inpatient, residential, outpatient, etc.) and what services had been received. In addition, parents were asked about their preferences for services. They were asked whether there was a strong preference for Hispanic-specific services, and to rank, in order of preference, issues that they felt should be key components of effective treatment (i.e., parenting, immigration/acculturation, drug counseling, and HIV-risk counseling).

### *Data Analyses*

Analyses were conducted in two steps. First, we investigated whether the hypothesized predictor variables predicted utilization in full sample, residential recommended sample only, and/or outpatient therapy recommended sample only (in that order) by entering each predictor into univariate logistical regression models for each sample. Next, those predictor variables that were significant ($p < .05$) were entered into a hierarchical logistic regression model for each sample type (full, residential, or outpatient). Checks for multicollinearity (i.e., when several predictors are highly correlated) among predictors indicated a high correlation ($r = -.70$) between two variables that were derived from a common measure (Parenting Practice-Discipline Avoidance and Parenting Practice-Discipline Effectiveness). As suggested by Pedhazur (1997), problems associated with multicollinearity were eliminated from the hierarchical regression analyses by creating a composite variable from the two highly correlated variables. The two variables were combined to a single variable, Parenting Effectiveness-Discipline Style that reflects parental discipline in terms of perceived efficacy and level of avoidance. The composite was created by reverse scoring Parenting Practice-Discipline Avoidance and summing it with Parenting Practice-Discipline Effectiveness. A high score on this composite reflects adaptive parenting (i.e., effective and low avoidance). Parenting Practice-Discipline Avoidance and Parenting Practice-Discipline Effectiveness were analyzed separately within the single predictor logistic regression analyses. The composite variable, Parenting Practices-Discipline Style, was used in the hierarchical regression analyses.

## *RESULTS*

### *Single Predictor Logistic Regression Models*

The single logistic regression analyses suggested a number of factors predicting general utilization of recommended therapeutic services (see Table 1).

TABLE 1. Predictors of Utilization: Results of the Univariate Logistic Regression Models

| | *Full Sample n = 86* | | | | | *Outpatient Sample n = 48* | | | | | *Residential Sample n = 38* | | | | |
|---|---|---|---|---|---|---|---|---|---|---|---|---|---|---|---|
| *Variable Name* | β | *SE* | *Odds Ratio* | *Wald Test* | *p-value* | β | *SE* | *Odds Ratio* | *Wald Test* | *p-value* | β | *SE* | *Odds Ratio* | *Wald Test* | *p-value* |
| Adolescent Psychopathology-Parent Report | | | | | | | | | | | | | | | |
| DISC-Externalizing Behaviors | −.37 | .18 | 0.58 | 4.19 | .04 | −.57 | .32 | .49 | 3.10 | .08 | −.22 | .24 | .76 | .82 | .37 |
| Parenting Practices-Parent Report | | | | | | | | | | | | | | | |
| Discipline Effectiveness | .63 | .27 | 1.77 | 5.57 | .02 | 1.34 | .50 | 2.15 | 7.11 | .01 | .23 | .34 | 1.23 | .49 | .49 |
| Discipline Avoidance | −.69 | .25 | 0.51 | 7.50 | .01 | −.85 | .37 | .55 | 5.33 | .02 | −.47 | .36 | .71 | 1.66 | .20 |
| Family Stress Indicators-Parent Report | | | | | | | | | | | | | | | |
| Parenting Stress-HSI | −.27 | .12 | 0.54 | 4.87 | .03 | −.18 | .17 | .71 | 1.04 | .31 | −.36 | .18 | .50 | 4.09 | .04 |

Parenting Practice-Discipline Avoidance ($p < .01$), Parenting Practice-Discipline Effectiveness ($p < .05$), Total Number of Adolescent Externalizing Disorders-Parent Report ($p < .05$), and HSI-Parenting Stress ($p < .05$) significantly predicted utilization of any recommendation type (i.e., outpatient or residential). Parenting Practice-Discipline Avoidance ($p < .05$), Parenting Practice-Discipline Effectiveness ($p < .01$) significantly predicted utilization in the outpatient-recommended sample and Parental Years in U.S. was included in the equation because of its conceptual value although it was only marginally significant (.07). HSI-Parenting Stress ($p < .05$) significantly predicted utilization in the residential-recommended sample. No other significant predictors were found at the univariate level. Mean differences between groups on key variables are presented in Figures 1-5.

Odds ratios were calculated to illustrate the relative magnitude of these effects. Odds ratios were calculated by comparing a standard deviation above to a standard deviation below the mean. For the full sample, parents who reported their child had more total externalizing behavior disorders were approximately half as likely to utilize recommended general therapy services.

Parents in the full sample who also reported more perceived discipline effectiveness were almost two times more likely to utilize therapy services, while those who endorsed more discipline avoidance were about half as likely to utilize these services. Parents who reported higher levels of parenting stress were also about half as likely to make use of therapy services.

FIGURE 1. Utilizer and Non-Utilizer Differences on Parent Discipline Style (Full Sample)

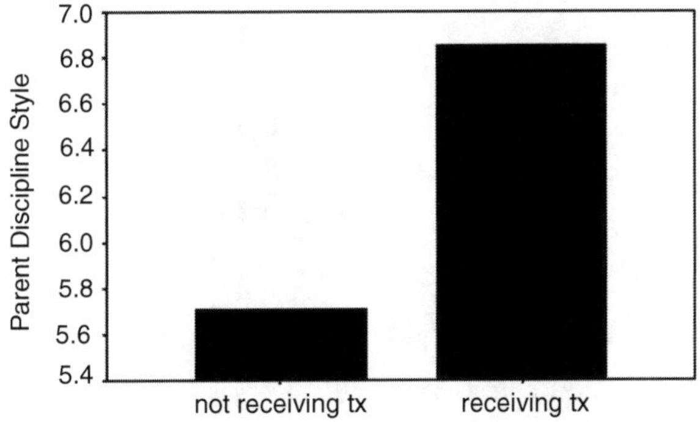

In the outpatient-recommended sample, parents who similarly reported more perceived discipline effectiveness were almost three times more likely to utilize therapy services, while those who endorsed more discipline avoidance were half as likely to utilize these services. Parents who reported more years in the United States were one and one-half times more likely to utilize recommended outpatient services.

In the residential-recommended sample, parents who reported experiencing more parenting stress were about half as likely to utilize residential services for their child than other parents.

FIGURE 2. Utilizer and Non-Utilizer Differences on Adolescent Externalizing Disorder (Full Sample)

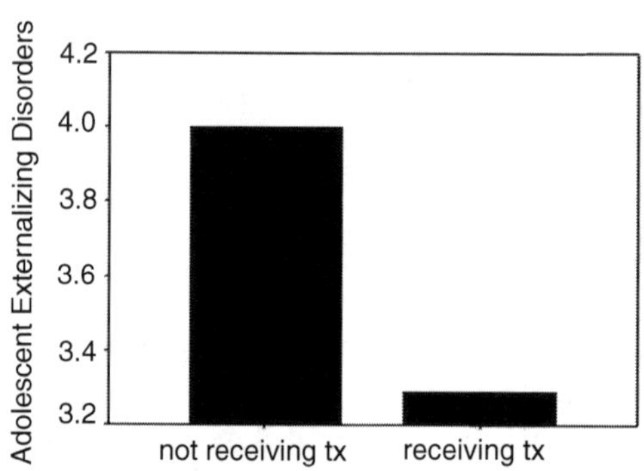


FIGURE 3. Utilizer and Non-Untilizer Differences on Parental Years in U.S. (Outpatient Sample)

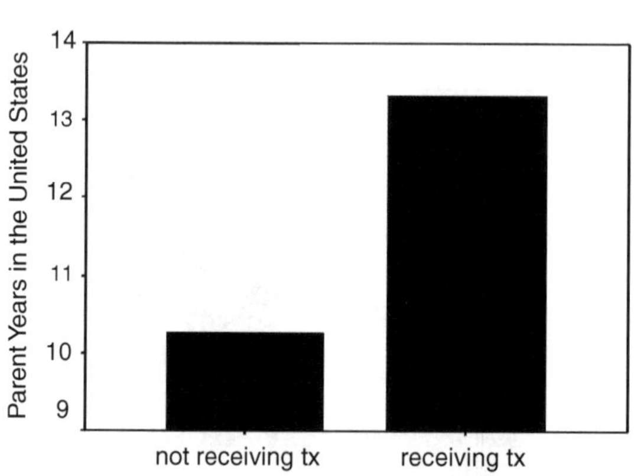

FIGURE 4. Utilizer and Non-Utilizer Differences on Parent Discipline Style (Outpatient Sample)

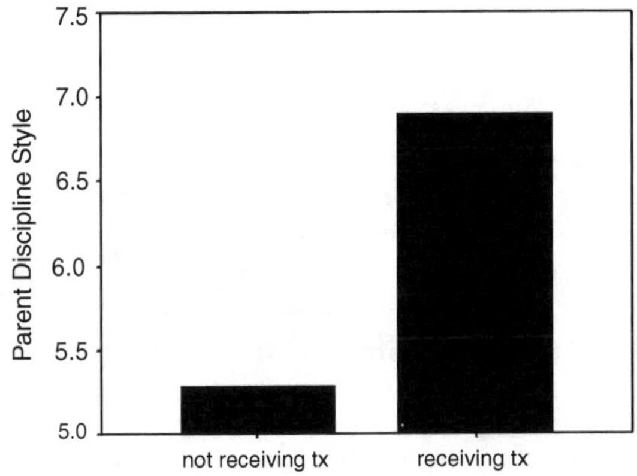


FIGURE 5. Utilizer and Non-Utilizer Differences on Parenting Stress (Residential Sample)

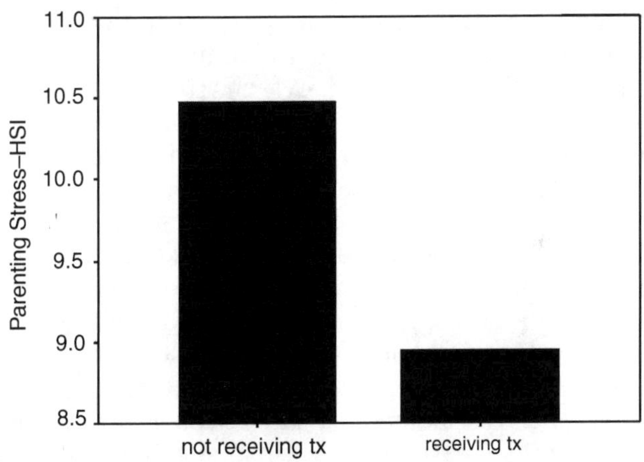


## *HIERARCHICAL LOGISTIC REGRESSION ANALYSES*

*Full sample.* In the hierarchical logistic regression analysis conducted with the full sample, the following predictors were entered as separate, sequential blocks: (a) total number of adolescent externalizing disorders-parent report, (b) Parenting Practices-Discipline Style, (c) HIS-

Parenting Stress. The first block, total number of adolescent externalizing disorders-parent report, significantly predicted utilization ($\chi^2$ = 4.18, $df$ = 1, $p < .05$). The second block, Parenting Practices-Discipline Style, significantly predicted utilization ($\chi^2$ = 8.73, $df$ = 2, $p < .05$), even after the variance due to total number of adolescent externalizing disorders was removed ($\chi^2$ = 4.54, $df$ = 1, $p < .05$). The third block, Parenting Stress, failed to significantly predict utilization (p > .05). However, the overall hypothesized model, including all 3 predictors: total number of adolescent externalizing disorders and Parenting Practices-Discipline Style and Parenting Stress did predict utilization ($\chi^2$ = 9.90, $df$ = 3, $p <$ .01). Therefore, the variance due to parental stress and total number of adolescent externalizing disorders-parent report and Parenting Practices- Discipline Style, affected the level of univariate significance that Parental Stress contributed to the prediction of utilization of recommended treatment. That is, the effect of Parenting Stress on utilization is mediated by the total number of adolescent externalizing disorders (parent report), and Parenting Practices-Discipline Style. The full model correctly predicts 63% of the cases.

*Outpatient sample.* The following two predictors were entered as separate, sequential blocks in the hierarchical logistic regression analysis conducted with the outpatient-recommended services sample: (a) Parenting Practices-Discipline Style and (b) Parental Years in the United States. Given the cultural salience of the latter variable as well as its marginal univariate significance ($p < .07$), it was included in the outpatient hierarchical regression analysis. The first block, Parenting Practices-Discipline Style, significantly predicted utilization ($\chi^2$ = 7.99, $df$ = 1, $p < .01$). The second block or full model, including Parenting Practices-Discipline Style and parent years in the United States, significantly predicted utilization ($\chi^2$ = 6.83, $df$ = 2, $p < .05$), even after the variance due to Parenting Practices-Discipline Style was removed ($\chi^2$ = 4.36, $df$ = 1, $p < .05$). The full model correctly predicts 81.3 % of the cases.

*Residential sample.* No hierarchical regression analyses were conducted due to findings suggesting a single, significant variable from the assessments used in the current study (i.e., parenting stress-HSI) ($\chi^2$ = 4.03, $df$ = 1, $p < .05$). The model correctly predicts 63.2% of the cases.

### *Correspondence Between Variables Predicting Utilization and Parent Treatment Preferences*

A set of exploratory analyses were conducted to attempt to shed light on the relationship of the predictor variables to two important questions asked during the follow-up interview: one asking about their preference for treatment specifically designed for Hispanics, and a second asking them to rank the importance of certain therapy themes (parenting practices, immigration/acculturation, drug counseling, and HIV-risk). Because the original analyses yielded a marginally significant difference on Parental Years in the United States in the outpatient sample, a median split (based on outpatient sample) of parent years in the United States was performed to distinguish between two groups: parents who spent 15 or less years in the United States (low) and parents who spent 16 or more years in the United States (high). Parental differences in years in the U.S. were significantly associated with reporting a preference of therapy addressing Hispanic specific issues among the outpatient sample ($k = -.38$, $p < .01$). That is, the group with fewer years in the U.S. was more likely to prefer a therapy specifically designed or tailored to Hispanic issues.

Because analyses showed (a) Parent Discipline Style significantly predicted utilization in the full sample, (b) Parent Discipline Style significantly predicted utilization of outpatient services, and (c) Parenting Stress predicted utilization of residential services, analyses were conducted to examine the correspondence between these variables and parental preferences in terms of therapy themes. A median split of Parent Discipline Style was performed to distinguish between two groups: parents scoring 8.22 or less (low parent discipline style) and parents scoring greater than 8.22 (high parent discipline style) across the full sample, and parents scoring 8.07 or less (low parent discipline style) and parents scoring greater than 8.07 (high parent discipline style) across the outpatient sample. Differences in level of Parent Discipline Style scores were not significantly associated with reporting a preference of therapy addressing parenting practice among full sample ($k = -.07$, *ns*). There was a significant association between Parent Discipline style differences and parent reporting preference of therapy addressing parenting practice among outpatient sample ($k = .33$, $p < .05$). That is, the more effective the parents reported their Discipline Style, the more likely they expressed a preference for therapy that addressed parenting issues.

A median split of Parenting Stress was conducted for the residential sample to address the significant findings. High parenting stress respondents indicated a score greater than 10, and low parenting stress parents reported a score of 10 or less. Differences between these two groups were significantly associated with reporting preference of therapy addressing parenting practice among residential sample ($k = .46$, $p < .05$).

That is, the more stress parents reported experiencing, the more likely they wanted therapy addressing parenting issues.

## DISCUSSION

The current study investigated the predictive impact of psychiatric, family, and ethnicity-related factors on the utilization of recommended substance abuse services. Analyses yielded a number of noteworthy findings with important implications for the clinical engagement of drug abusing Hispanic adolescents into treatment. Adolescents and families who utilized various types of recommended therapy services were distinguished from non-utilizing families by several key factors that were the focus of this study.

The first interesting finding was that a parenting practice style characterized by involved parents who did not avoid disciplining issues and felt effective and competent in their parenting were most likely to seek services overall (residential + outpatient), and separately among the subsample for whom outpatient treatment was recommended. This along with low externalizing behavior and low parental stress were associated with higher utilization. On the flip side, parents who feel ineffective, who avoid disciplinary actions, who have youth with multiple externalizing behaviors, and feel high levels of parenting stress are less likely to engage. Interestingly, it appears that a high level of parental stress level does not seem to impact utilization likelihood alone; but rather, is mediated by the number of externalizing problems adolescents exhibit and the parenting discipline style carried out by parents. The findings regarding parental characteristics and externalizing behaviors do not bode well for those families most in need of services. One would hope that the more (a) externalizing problems adolescents exhibit, and the more (b) parents report problems in their parenting skills and levels of stress (problems that could be addressed via parenting and mental health interventions), the more families would utilize recommended services. However, the opposite appears to be occurring among Hispanic drug abusing populations. This finding is consistent with our previous work pointing to the need for specialized engagement interventions developed to engage adolescents and families most in need, into services (Santisteban & Szapocznik, 1994; Santisteban et al., 1996; Szapocznik et al., 1988).

Worthy of additional discussion is the finding that high symptomatology is associated with diminished utilization. In some ways, this is contrary to much of the available literature. Our hypothesis is that the findings of studies investigating the relationship between level of symptomatology and service utilization may differ substantially depending on the overall level of functioning of the sample. That is, studies of non-clinical samples may find a positive relationship between adolescent and parent symptomatology and utilization because some level of problem history may increase the "readiness" for services. However, in a sample consisting fully of clinical cases with high levels of symptomatology, one may find that those with the highest levels of symptoms are actually hindered from utilizing services. In these clinical samples one may find the opposite effect or a negative association between symptoms and utilization. If this is true, we would expect a reverse U-shaped curve for the relationship between symptoms and utilization if cases at all ranges (clinical and non-clinical) were investigated together. Interestingly, the same pattern of association between symptoms and utilization was also evident in that high parenting stress led to less utilization of residential treatment. This is also counter-intuitive because anecdotally one often thinks that highly stressed families may seek to "fix the problem" by taking the youth out of the home and placing them in residential treatment. Even this process, however, appears to be hindered by high levels of stress.

It is also important to note those variables that might have been expected to, but did not, predict service utilization in this study. For example, none of the family composition and demographic factors previously thought to impact service utilization (family size, gender, income) were found to predict utilization in this study. Parental years in the U.S. was only marginally predictive variable, with those in the U.S. longer showing greater utilization. Of the key demographic variables, one–family income–may not have received an adequate test because of the very restricted range in this sample.

## *LIMITATIONS*

Several limitations concerning these studies should be noted. First, the study analyzed a limited sample of adolescents referred to treatment for their drug abuse and related externalizing problems. Generalizability limitations in terms of adolescents referred for psychiatric problems outside the scope of the current study are important to note. The ability of certain factors to predict utilization may not generalize to other types of adolescents and families. Future research is required to assess whether these predictors would identify utilizing from non-utilizing adolescents recommended treatment for additional psychiatric conditions.

Second, the sample is entirely composed of Hispanic adolescents and their families. Although research on underserved populations such as the one sampled in the current sample is valuable to fill the void in the literature (Nagayama Hall, 2001), the findings could be unique to specific sample characteristics.

Third, there were additional possible predictors of utilization that were not studied (e.g., readiness for therapy factors). Past treatment service research (see Dakof, Tejeda, & Liddle, 2001 for review) have described multiple reasons for non-utilization of therapy including (a) adolescents' motivation and readiness (Melnick, De Leon, Hawke, Jainchill, & Kressel, 1997), (b) parents' belief that the treatment will not help, (c) parent-therapist relationship, and (d) practical obstacles to treatment (Kazdin, Holland, & Crowley, 1997). It would be helpful to continue to investigate these important predictors of utilization of treatment.

Finally, the interviews that collected service utilization data were conducted six weeks following discharge and, therefore, it is not known whether some families may have followed the treatment recommendations after the interview. Although we believe that it is unlikely that many families would initiate a continuation of services if they had not already, it would be helpful to investigate this possibility directly.

## *CLINICAL IMPLICATIONS*

The results of this study emphasize the need for specialized engagement interventions that can offset the power of key psychiatric and parenting factors that serve as obstacles to engagement into treatment. The expectations that highly clinical families, especially those in most need, can organize themselves to meet the challenge of negotiating their way through the treatment systems and engage into treatment, appears unrealistic.

It is important for both ends of the service delivery system (i.e., discharge and referral systems, and receiving substance abuse and mental health providers) to understand how maladaptive parenting style and high levels of symptomatology will keep youth and families from much needed services. It is also important to note that both parental and adolescent factors are predictive. Family factors and family-member role in service utilization cannot be understated, especially when speaking of child and adolescent service utilization. Future research may be able to focus on ways of screening for specific factors that lead to non-utilization and the development of specific engagement strategies tailored to those family characteristics.

## REFERENCES

Armsden, G. C., & Greenberg, M. T. (1987). The Inventory of Parent and Peer Attachment: Relationships to well-being in adolescence. *Journal of Youth & Adolescence, 16*(5), 427-454.

Cervantes, R. C., Padilla, A. M., & Salgado de Snyder, N. (1991). The Hispanic stress inventory: A culturally relevant approach to psychosocial assessment. *Psychological Assessment: A Journal of Consulting & Clinical Psychology, 3*(3), 438-447.

Cornelius, J. R., Pringle, J., Jernigan, J., Kirisci, L., & Clark, D. B. (2001). Correlates of mental health service utilization and unmet need among a sample of male adolescents. *Addictive Behaviors, 26*, 11-19.

Dakof, G., Tejeda, M., & Liddle, H. (2001). Predictors of engagement in adolescent drug abuse treatment. *Journal of the American Academy of Child & Adolescent Psychiatry, 40*, 274-281.

Farmer, E. M., Burns, B. J., Angold, A., & Costello, E. J. (1997). Impact of children's mental health problems on families: Relationships with services use. *Journal of Emotional & Behavioral Disorders, 5*, 230-238.

Goodman, S. H., Lahey, B. B., Fielding, B., Dulcan, M., Narrow, W., & Regier, D. (1997). Representativeness of clinical samples of youths with mental disorders: A preliminary population based study. *Journal of Abnormal Psychology, 106,* 3-14.

Gorman-Smith, D., Tolan, P. H., Zelli, A., & Huesmann, L. R. (1996). The relation of family functioning to violence among inner-city minority youths. *Journal of Family Psychology, 10*, 115-129.

Hough, R. L., Hazen, A. L., Soriano, F. I., Wood, P., McCabe, K., & Yeh, M. (2002). Mental health services for Latino adolescents with psychiatric disorders. *Psychiatric Services, 53*, 1556-1562.

Johnson, S. D., Stiffman, A., Hadley-Ives, E., & Elze, D. (2001). An analysis of stressors and co-morbid mental health problems that contribute to youths' paths to substance specific services. *Journal of Behavioral Health Services & Research, 28*, 412-426.

Kazdin, A. E., Holland, L., & Crowley, M. (1997). Family experience of barriers to treatment and premature termination from child therapy. *Journal of Consulting & Clinical Psychology, 65*, 453-463.

Loeber, R., Stouthamer-Loeber, M., Van Kammen, W., & Farrington, D. P. (1991). Initiation, escalation and desistance in juvenile offending and their correlates. *Journal of Criminal Law & Criminology, 82*, 36-82.

Logan, D. E., & King, C. A. (2001). Parental facilitation of adolescent mental health service utilization: A conceptual and empirical review. *Clinical Psychology: Science and Practice*, *3*, 319-333.

Lucas, C. P., Zhang, H., Fisher, P. W., Shaffer, D., Regier, D. A., Narrow, W. E., Bourdon, K., Dulcan, M. K., Canino, G., Rubio-Stipec, M., Lahey, B. B., & Friman, P. (2001). The DISC Predictive Scale (DPS): Efficiently screening for diagnoses. *Journal of the American Academy of Child & Adolescent Psychiatry*, *40*, 443-449.

Melnick, G., De Leon, G., Hawke, J., Jainchill, N., & Kressel, D. (1997). Motivation and readiness for therapeutic community treatment among adolescents and adult substance abusers. *American Journal of Drug & Alcohol Abuse*, *23*, 485-506.

Nagayama Hall, G. C. (2001). Psychotherapy research with ethnic minorities: Empirical, ethical, and conceptual issues. *Journal of Consulting & Clinical Psychology*, *69*, 502-510.

Pedhazur, E. J. (1997). *Multiple regression in behavioral research: Explanation and prediction* (3rd Edition). Harcourt Brace.

Pumariega, A. J., Glover, S., Holzer, C. E., & Nguyen, H. (1998). Utilization of mental health services in a tri-ethnic sample of adolescents. *Community Mental Health Journal*, *34,* 145-156.

Rogler, L. H. (1998). Research on mental health services for Hispanics. In P. B. Organista, K. M. Chun, & G. Marin (Eds.), *Readings in ethnic psychology* (pp. 311-323). New York: Routledge.

Santisteban, D.A., & Szapocznik, J. (1994) Bridging theory research and practice to more successfully engage substance abusing youth and their families into therapy. *Journal of Child & Adolescent Substance Abuse*, *32*(2), 9-24.

Santisteban, D. A., Szapocznik, J., Perez-Vidal, A., Kurtines, W., Murray, E. J., & LaPerriere, A. (1996). Efficacy of Interventions for engaging Youth/Families into treatment and the some variables that may contribute to differential effectiveness. *Journal of Family Psychology*, *10*(1), 35-44.

Substance Abuse and Mental Health Services Administration (2002). National Survey on Drug Use and Health.

Szapocznik, J., Kurtines, W. M., & Fernandez, T. (1980). Bicultural involvement and adjustment in Hispanic-American youths. *International Journal of Intercultural Relations*, *4*, 353-365.

Szapocznik, J., Perez-Vidal, A., Brickman, A. L., Foote, F. H., Santisteban, D., Hervis, O., & Kurtines, W. M. (1988). Engaging adolescents drug abusers and their families into treatment: A strategic structural systems approach. *Journal of Consulting & Clinical Psychology*, *56*(4), 552-557.

Szapocznik, J., Scopetta, M., Kurtines, W., & Arnalde, M. A. (1978). Theory and measurement of acculturation. *Interamerican Journal of Psychology*, *12*, 113-130.

Takeuchi, D. T., Sue, S., & Yeh, M. (1998). Return rates and outcomes from ethnicity specific mental health programs in Los Angeles. In Organista, P.B., Chun, K.M., & Marin, G. (1998). *Readings in ethnic psychology* (324-334). New York: Routledge.

The National Advisory Mental Health Council Workgroup on Child and Adolescent Mental Health Intervention Development and Deployment. (2001). Blueprint for Change: Research on Child and Adolescent Mental Health. Washington, DC.

Winters, K. C., & Henly, G. A. (1989). *Personal Experiences Inventory*. Los Angeles, CA: Western Psychological Services.

Wu, P., Hoven, C. W., & Fuller, C. J. (2003). Factors associated with adolescents receiving drug treatment: Findings from the National Household Survey on Drug Abuse. *Journal of Behavioral Health Services & Research, 30*, 190-201.

Wu, P., Hoven, C. W., Tiet, Q., Kovalenko, P.,; & Wicks, J. (2002). Factors associated with adolescent utilization of alcohol treatment services. *American Journal of Drug & Alcohol Abuse, 28,* 353-369.

Zwaanswijk, M., Van der Ende, J., Verhaak, P., Bensing, J. M., & Verhulst, F. C. (2003). Factors associated with adolescent mental health service need and utilization. *Journal of the American Academy of Child & Adolescent Psychiatry, 42*, 692-700.

# Factors Associated with Drug Treatment Entry Patterns Among Hispanic Women Injection Drug Users Seeking Treatment

Lena M. Lundgren
Hortensia Amaro
Linsey Ben-Ami

**SUMMARY.** This paper examines patterns of drug treatment entry and factors that are associated with these patterns among 1,849 Hispanic women injection drug users (IDUs). The data analyzed originates from a statewide drug-treatment database covering seven years, 1996-2002. Through the use of logistic regression analyses, the study identified

Lena M. Lundgren, PhD, is Associate Professor, School of Social Work, Boston University (E-mail: llundgre@bu.edu). Hortensia Amaro, PhD, is Distinguished Professor and Director, Institute on Urban Health Research, Northeastern University (E-mail: h.amaro@neu.edu). Linsey Ben-Ami, MPH, is Research Assistant, Center on Work and Family, School of Social Work, Boston University (E-mail: lbenami@bu.edu).

The assistance of Michael Botticelli, Theresa Anderson, PhD, and Mitzi Knepper, MSW, from the Bureau is gratefully acknowledged.

This study was funded by grant # H-79TI12241-01 from the Center for Substance Abuse Treatment (CSAT) through a subcontract with the Massachusetts Bureau of Substance Abuse Services.

[Haworth co-indexing entry note]: "Factors Associated with Drug Treatment Entry Patterns Among Hispanic Women Injection Drug Users Seeking Treatment." Lundgren, Lena M., Hortensia Amaro, and Linsey Ben-Ami. Co-published simultaneously in *Journal of Social Work Practice in the Addictions* (The Haworth Press, Inc.) Vol. 5, No. 1/2, 2005, pp. 157-174; and: *Substance Abusing Latinos: Current Research on Epidemiology, Prevention, and Treatment* (ed: Mario R. De La Rosa, Lori K. Holleran, and Shulamith Lala Ashenberg Straussner) The Haworth Press, Inc., 2005, pp. 157-174. Single or multiple copies of this article are available for a fee from The Haworth Document Delivery Service [1-800-HAWORTH, 9:00 a.m. - 5:00 p.m. (EST). E-mail address: docdelivery@haworthpress.com].

http://www.haworthpress.com/web/JSWPA

Digital Object Identifier: 10.1300/J160v05n01_08

significant differences in predisposing, need and enabling factors in the use of detoxification only, residential treatment, or methadone maintenance. Compared to other Hispanics, Puerto Rican women were 40 percent less likely to use only detoxification services and one and a half times more likely to use methadone maintenance. Having health insurance was an especially important factor associated with methadone treatment utilization. Two of the most important factors associated with residential treatment use were history of mental health services utilization and involvement with the criminal justice system. This article discusses specific social work practice implications including the need for social work practitioners to promote services such as residential treatment, to be trained in treatment of co-occurring mental health disorders, especially among women in residential treatment, and the need to establish close linkages with the mental health and criminal justice systems. 

**KEYWORDS.** Hispanic women, drug-treatment utilization, injection drug use

## *INTRODUCTION*

Heroin use has increased dramatically in Massachusetts over the past five years. Indicators of this include the rise of heroin mentions in the emergency room and the increase of people seeking substance abuse treatment who report previous heroin use. In Boston alone, the number of emergency department mentions of heroin reported by the Drug Abuse Warning Network (DAWN) rose from 2,738 in 1998 to 3,999 in 2002 (SAMHSA, 2003a). Among all women receiving substance abuse treatment at state licensed treatment centers the number reporting heroin use in the past year rose from 23% in 1992 to 44.6% in 2002 (MDPH, 2003).

This increase in heroin use is closely associated with the increase in the number of injection drug use related HIV cases in the state. In Massachusetts, 35% of persons with HIV/AIDS were exposed to the virus through injection drug use, while in the U.S. overall, 25% of persons with HIV/AIDS contracted the disease through injection drug use. Currently, injection drug use is the second leading source of the spread of the HIV virus in the state (KFF, 2002).

According to the most recent NHSDA, Hispanics show the highest rates for illicit drug abuse or dependence (SAMHSA, 2002a). Further, the rise in heroin use noted in the U.S. has been especially pronounced among young Hispanic adults (Frank, 2000) resulting in injection drug use accounting for 36% of diagnosed AIDS cases among Hispanic men and 38% among Hispanic women (CDC, 2002). Further, HIV seroprevalence is higher among Puerto Ricans compared to other Hispanics (Diaz, Buehler, Castro, & Ward,1993; NIDA, 1992; Selik, Castro, & Pappaioanou, 1989; Selik, Castro, & Pappaioanou, 1988) and injection drug use plays a predominant role in HIV infection among Puerto Ricans compared to other Hispanic groups (COSSMHO, 1991). Similar to drug use rates among Hispanics overall, drug use among Hispanic women varies by Hispanic group with a higher percentage of Puerto Rican women reporting past month use than other Hispanic women (Amaro, Whitaker, Coffman, & Heeren, 1990; SAMHSA, 2002b).

Consistent with rates of opiate use, national data on treatment admissions indicate that opiates are the most common primary substance of abuse among treatment admissions (34%) in Hispanic women (SAM HSA, 2002b). The 1999 Treatment Episode Data Set (TEDS) documented differences in patterns of drug treatment admissions among Hispanics compared to non-Hispanic Whites wherein Hispanics had a larger percentage of admissions for opiate abuse (32%) compared to non-Hispanics (15%) (SAMHSA, 2002b). Robles et al. (2003) found significant variations in the use of drug treatment services among Puerto Ricans residing in the continental U.S. and Puerto Rico. Also, use of all drug treatment modalities, with the exception of outpatient treatment, was lower among Puerto Ricans living in New York City compared to those in Puerto Rico (Robles et al., 2003). A study of treatment use in Massachusetts found that Hispanics, who were primarily Puerto Rican, were less likely than non-Hispanic Whites to enter residential treatment (Lundgren, Amodeo, Ferguson, & Davis, 2001). However, previous studies have not investigated patterns of drug treatment use among Hispanic women. We were specifically interested in patterns of drug treatment use among Hispanic women because they comprise the largest racial/ethnic minority group in the U.S. (U.S. Bureau of the Census, 2003). In Massachusetts, opiate related overdoses have increased (MDPH, 2004) and the drug treatment admissions for opiate abuse have increased for Hispanic women (Lundgren & Ben-Ami, 2003).

The aim of this study was to investigate the patterns of drug treatment entry among Hispanic women heroin users and to identify factors that account for differences in drug treatment entry patterns. Specifically, the study explored factors associated with the likelihood to enter either (1) detoxification only, a treatment modality known to have limited success if not used in combination with other modalities, or to also use (2) residential treatment or (3) methadone treatment, modalities more likely to result in abstinence and reduced HIV risk behaviors. This type of information is critical in order to develop culturally competent drug treatment recommendations for Hispanic women.

The conceptual framework of the study effort is based on a behavioral health model Andersen (1995) and Aday and Awe (1997). This "health services utilization" model integrates an array of correlates of health and health care behaviors from sociology, psychology, economics, and medicine into predisposing, enabling and need predictors of the "use of physician, hospital, and dentist services" (Aday & Awe, 1997, p. 153). Here, we are expanding this model to include substance abuse treatment. In this model, characteristics such as age, race/ethnicity, homelessness and parental status are termed "immutable" or predisposing. Whereas health policy responses cannot change such attributes, these characteristics need to be acknowledged as they often "define target groups at greater risk of illness or poorer access to care" (Aday & Awe, 1997, p. 160). Based on the Anderson framework, the study also considered the following enabling factors: health-insurance status, mental health service use, involvement in the criminal justice system, number of times having used the drug-treatment system, and employment status. Specifically, having health insurance can affect the type of treatment used. For example, privately run residential programs often require health insurance. Mental health service use and criminal justice involvement is here defined as enabling in that both systems provide either referrals or mandate participation in drug treatment. Similarly, previous drug-treatment use is often a predictor of future drug-treatment use (Hser, Grella, Shih-Chao, Anglin, & Brown, 1999; Robles et al., 2003). Employment is defined as enabling in that it, in some circumstances, provides access to health insurance. Finally, the study considered level of drug use as a measure of drug treatment need.

## *METHODS*

Patterns of drug treatment entry for Hispanic women IDUs residing in Massachusetts were examined for a seven year time period, 1996-2002. Specifically, three logistic regression models were developed to examine whether the following factors were associated with the likelihood of entering only detoxification compared to methadone maintenance, or residential treatment:

a. Pre-disposing characteristics: ethnicity, age, education, homelessness, and parental status.
b. Enabling factors: health-insurance status, mental health service use, involvement in the criminal justice system, number of times having used the drug-treatment system and employment status.
c. Need: level of drug use (having injected drugs in the past month).

The above relationships were examined for a group of 1,849 women who entered drug treatment in the commonwealth of Massachusetts between 1996-2002 and who reported having injected drugs in the year prior to treatment entry.

## *SOURCE OF DATA AND SAMPLE*

Data for this study were collected as part of the Massachusetts Bureau of Substance Abuse Services (BSAS) Management Information System (MIS), which is comprised of information collected at all admissions to substance abuse treatment programs licensed by BSAS. The BSAS Management Information System database has been recognized as one of the relatively few state-wide drug treatment databases which is both comprehensive and accurate enough to permit detailed exploration of drug treatment utilization (McCarty, McGuire, Harwood, & Field, 1998). The MIS database is a claims-based system and payment cannot be made without accurate and comprehensive admissions information (McCarty et al., 1998). The database was originally organized by admission date and each time a client was admitted the individual would receive a new entry with a unique identifier. Each client had a mean of 5.9 entries, one per every admission into substance abuse treatment services.

The study population consists of 1,849 women who reported their ethnicity as Hispanic/Latino, were between the ages of 18 and 75, reported injecting drugs in the year prior to any admission and who had at least one admission to a state licensed substance abuse treatment program between 1996-2002. The primary drug used was heroin.

## *MEASUREMENTS*

The first step in the analysis was to condense each individual's admission entries into one client level entry. In order to perform this step, it was necessary to recode some of the original variables into summary variables.

Ethnicity was coded according to self-report at first admission. Among the study sample, over two thirds (70.6%) reported their ethnicity as Puerto Rican. Other groups included Central American (21.0%), Dominican (1.7%), Mexican (0.8%), Cuban (0.5%) or other Hispanic (5.5%). For the logistic regression analyses all categories of Hispanic ethnicity besides Puerto Rican were collapsed into one group in order to increase the robustness of the analyses.

Age was coded as the mean age across all treatment admissions. Education was recoded from the original BSAS continuous variable into three categories: less than high school, high school graduate and more than high school, based on highest number of years of education reported across all admissions. Homelessness was coded as having ever reported being homeless at any treatment admission. Employment was coded as having ever been employed, full or part-time, at any treatment admission.

Severity of drug use was measured using the variable "injected in the past month" vs. "did not inject in the past month." Women who had injected within the month prior to their last treatment admission were coded as "injected in the past month." This variable was the most reliable for measuring level of drug use, given the limitations within the dataset. Parental status was self-reported at all admissions and was coded as a three-category variable. The categories were as follows: not a parent; reported having children (under the age of 18) but not residing with them at any treatment admission; and reported residing with their children at any treatment admission.

The health insurance variable originally comprised three categories: (1) no health insurance, (2) public health insurance, and (3) private health insurance. Health insurance status was recoded as a three-category variable: having never reported having health insurance at any admission; reporting having public health insurance at any admission, but never reporting private health insurance; ever reporting private health insurance at any admission. Mental health treatment was coded as ever reporting having received mental health treatment. Mental health treatment included receiving either outpatient counseling or having been hospitalized one or more times for a mental health problem.

The criminal justice variable was a measure of whether women had ever self-reported currently receiving services from the Department of Corrections, Office of the Commissioner of Probation and/or the Massachusetts Parole Board at the time of any admission.

## *DEPENDENT VARIABLES*

The first variable, "detoxification only," measures whether an IDU had ever been admitted to a detoxification program in Massachusetts between 1996-2002, and to no other treatment modality. The second variable "residential treatment," measures whether an IDU was ever admitted to a residential treatment program in Massachusetts between 1996 and 2002. The third variable measures whether a client was ever admitted to methadone treatment between 1996 and 2002.

## *DATA ANALYSIS*

The patterns of drug treatment entry for Hispanic IDUs were examined for a seven year time period, 1996-2002. Bi-variate analysis was conducted to describe populations and differences in entry into methadone, residential treatment and detoxification only. Since the majority of the variables were highly inter-correlated, logistic regression methods were utilized to untangle the relationships between variables. Specifically, three logistic regression models were developed to examine factors associated with differences in the likelihood of entering only detoxification compared to methadone maintenance or residential treatment, controlling for predisposing (i.e., Hispanic ethnicity, age, parental status), enabling (i.e., health-insurance status, mental health service use, involvement in the criminal justice system, number of times having used the drug-treatment system and employment status), and need (level of drug use) factors.

Binomial logistic regression was used to examine the associations between the independent variables and each of the types of treatment outcomes of concern. In each model, the variables were entered in a single block. Criterion categories among the categorical independent variables are indicated showing the odds-ratio results.

## *RESULTS*

As evidenced in Table 1, the majority of Hispanic women were Puerto Rican (70.6%). The remaining 29.4% reported their ethnicity as: Central American (21.0%), Dominican (1.7%), Mexican (0.8%), Cuban (0.5%) or other Hispanic (5.5%). Close to 80% of the women had a high-school degree or less. About a third (36.1%) reported being homeless. More than 80% of the women were parents, but only approximately half of these parents reported residing with their children at the time of drug-treatment admission. Seventy percent had public health insurance and 17.2% never had insurance at any of their drug treatment admissions. Less than one third of Hispanic women receiving drug treatment in Massachusetts (27.2%) reported receiving services through the criminal justice system when they entered drug treatment. Approximately 60% reported having received mental health services. The majority (79.3%) of these women, who all reported having injected drugs in the past year, also reported having injected drugs in the past month prior to treatment entry.

Twenty-five percent of the women had used only detoxification services between 1996 and 2002. Approximately 27% of the population had entered residential treatment and approximately 48% of these women had entered methadone maintenance services between 1996 and 2002.

## *LOGISTIC REGRESSION RESULTS*

As Tables 2-4 indicate, a number of predisposing, enabling and need factors were significantly associated with utilization of drug treatment services. Model 1 presented in Table 2 shows that predisposing factors associated with using only detoxification services were being of other Hispanic background compared to Puerto Rican, having no children compared to those living with children, and not having a high school degree compared to those with a high school degree. Controlling for pre-

TABLE 1. Univariate Statistics (N = 1,849)

| **Variable** | **Percentage or Mean (SD)** |
|---|---|
| **Predisposing Factors** | |
| **Ethnicity** | |
| Puerto Rican | 70.6% |
| Other Hispanic | 29.4 |
| **Mean age in years** | 32.3(7.6) |
| **Level of Education** | |
| Less than high school | 43.0% |
| High school graduate | 36.6 |
| More than high school | 20.4 |
| **Homelessness** | |
| Reported being homeless at any intake | 36.1 |
| **Parental Status** | |
| No children at any intake | 17.7% |
| Lives apart from their children | 39.6 |
| Lives with their children | 42.7 |
| Mean number of children | 2.4(1.9) |
| **Enabling Factors** | |
| **Employment** | |
| Reported being employed full time, part-time or occasionally | 21.0 |
| **Health Insurance** | |
| No health insurance at any admission | 17.2% |
| Public health insurance | 71.0 |
| Private health insurance | 11.8 |
| **Mental Health** | |
| Ever received mental health treatment | 59.5% |
| **Criminal Justice** | |
| Reported receiving criminal justice services at any admission | 27.2% |
| **Drug Treatment** | |
| Mean number of treatments | 5.9(7.0) |
| **Need Factors** | |
| **Drug Use** | |
| **Reported injecting drugs in the month prior to any intake** | 79.3% |
| **Drug Treatment Modalities** | |
| Only entered detoxification services | 25.2% |
| Having entered residential treatment | 26.9 |
| Having entered methadone maintenance | 47.7 |

TABLE 2. Logistic Regression Characteristics Associated with Having Used Detoxification Services Only in Massachusetts BSAS Licensed Facilities (N = 1,849)

| Variable<br>**Predisposing Factors** | Odds Ratio | (95% CI: Lower, Upper) |
|---|---|---|
| **Ethnicity** | | |
| Puerto Rican** | .588 | (.414, .837) |
| Other Hispanic(a) | | |
| **Mean age in years** | .982 | (.964, 1.000) |
| **Level of Education** | | |
| Less than high school(a) | | |
| High school graduate* | 1.479 | (1.088, 2.011) |
| More than high school | 1.342 | (.846, 2.130) |
| **Homelessness** | | |
| Reported being homeless at any intake(b) | 1.277 | (.905, 1.803) |
| **Parental Status** | | |
| No children at any intake(a) | | |
| Lives apart from their children | .948 | (.600, 1.498) |
| Lives with their children** | .483 | (.296, .788) |
| Mean number of children | 1.047 | (.953, 1.149) |
| **Enabling Factors** | | |
| **Employment** | | |
| Reported being employed full time, part-time or occasionally(b)* | .567 | (.350, .917) |
| **Health Insurance** | | |
| No health insurance at any admission(a) | | |
| Public health insurance*** | .411 | (.295, .573) |
| Private health insurance | .771 | (.419, 1.416) |
| **Mental Health** | | |
| Ever received mental health treatment*** | .376 | (.280, .504) |
| **Criminal Justice** | | |
| Reported receiving criminal justice services at any admission(b)*** | .250 | (.144, .435) |
| **Drug Treatment** | | |
| Mean number of treatments*** | .723 | (.667, .783) |
| **Need Factors** | | |
| **Drug Use** | | |
| **Reported injecting drugs in the month prior to last intake***** | 8.929 | (5.319, 14.99) |

Model Chi Square $\chi^2 = 775.367$, df =15 , p < .000
Nagelkerke R Square = .506
(a) Reference group
(b) Yes group is compared to the no group
* p ≤.05, ** p ≤ .01, ***p ≤ .001

disposing factors, those least likely to utilize only detoxification services were those with health insurance, recent employment, history of mental health service utilization, more drug treatment entries, and criminal justice involvement. On the other hand, women most likely to use only detoxification treatment were those who reported injection drug use in the previous month. They were over eight times more likely than those who did not report recent injection drug use to have used only detoxification services and no other treatment modality.

Model 2 shown in Table 3 indicates that the predisposing factors associated with entering methadone treatment were being Puerto Rican, older age, and living with children, while those with a history of homelessness were less likely to enter methadone treatment. After controlling for predisposing factors, three enabling factors were significantly associated with use of methadone treatment. The factor most significantly associated with the use of methadone treatment use was health insurance status wherein those with private or public health insurance were six to seven times more likely to enter methadone treatment. Other enabling factors included having used mental health services and more drug treatment entries. Injection drug use in the last month was also significantly associated with using this treatment modality.

The third and final logistic regression model shown in Table 4 examined factors associated with the likelihood of having used residential drug treatment. This model shows that the predisposing factor of having been homeless was associated with a three-fold greater likelihood of entering residential treatment. After controlling for predisposing factors, women with a history of mental health service utilization or involvement with the criminal justice system were two times more likely than those without such histories to enter residential treatment. Those with a greater number of previous entries to drug treatment were also more likely to enter residential treatment.

## *DISCUSSION*

This article sought to identify patterns of drug treatment utilization among the population of Hispanic women who had utilized Massachusetts' drug treatment system. First, health insurance seems to be a critical factor associated with the use of detoxification only and methadone treatment, but not of residential treatment. Fewer women with health insurance than those with no health insurance used only detoxification services whereas those with health insurance were more likely to use

TABLE 3. Logistic Regression Characteristics Associated with Having Ever Used Methadone Maintenance in Massachusetts BSAS Licensed Facilities (N = 1,849)

| Predisposing Factors | Odds Ratio | (95% CI: Lower, Upper) |
|---|---|---|
| **Ethnicity** | | |
| Puerto Rican*** | 1.589 | (1.222, 2.068) |
| Other Hispanic(a) | | |
| **Mean age in years**** | 1.019 | (1.005, 1.034) |
| **Level of Education** | | |
| Less than high school(a) | | |
| High school graduate | .856 | (.668, 1.097) |
| More than high school | 1.036 | (.751, 1.430) |
| **Homelessness** | | |
| Reported being homeless at any intake(b)*** | .447 | (.344, .582) |
| **Parental Status** | | |
| No children at any intake(a) | | |
| Lives apart from their children | .999 | (.690, 1.446) |
| Lives with their children*** | 1.868 | (1.293, 2.699) |
| Mean number of children | 1.015 | (.945, 1.090) |
| **Enabling Factors** | | |
| **Employment** | | |
| Reported being employed full time, part-time or occasionally(b) | 1.195 | (.895, 1.595) |
| **Health Insurance** | | |
| No health insurance at any admission(a) | | |
| Public health insurance*** | 7.355 | (4.828, 11.202) |
| Private health insurance*** | 5.811 | (3.452, 9.782) |
| **Mental Health** | | |
| Ever received mental health treatment*** | 1.677 | (1.319, 2.133) |
| **Criminal Justice** | | |
| Reported receiving criminal justice services at any admission(b) | .766 | (.579, 1.013) |
| **Drug Treatment** | | |
| Mean number of treatments*** | 1.103 | (1.075, 1.131) |
| **Drug Use** | | |
| **Reported injecting drugs in the month prior to last intake***** | 1.660 | (1.276, 2.158) |

Model Chi Square $\chi^2 = 504.315$, df =15 , p < .000
Nagelkerke R Square .319
(a) Reference group
(b) Yes group is compared to the no group
p ≤.05, ** p ≤ .01, ***p ≤ .001

TABLE 4. Logistic Regression Characteristics Associated with Having Ever Used Residential Treatment in Massachusetts BSAS Licensed Facilities (N = 1,849)

| **Predisposing Factors** | Odds Ratio | (95% CI: Lower, Upper) |
|---|---|---|
| **Ethnicity** | | |
| Puerto Rican | .977 | (.728, 1.312) |
| Other Hispanic(a) | | |
| **Mean age in years*** | .980 | (.962, .998) |
| **Level of Education** | | |
| Less than high school(a) | | |
| High school graduate | 1.100 | (.811, 1.493) |
| More than high school | 1.421 | (.989, 2.042) |
| **Homelessness** | | |
| Reported being homeless at any intake(b)*** | 3.029 | (2.311, 3.971) |
| **Parental Status** | | |
| No children at any intake(a) | | |
| Lives apart from their children | .700 | (.457, 1.074) |
| Lives with their children | .770 | (.499, 1.187) |
| Mean number of children | 1.037 | (.952, 1.130) |
| **Enabling Factors** | | |
| **Employment** | | |
| Reported being employed full time, part-time or occasionally(b) | 1.290 | (.941, 1.769) |
| **Health Insurance** | | |
| No health insurance at any admission(a) | | |
| Public health insurance | 1.035 | (.685, 1.564) |
| Private health insurance | 1.124 | (.659, 1.917) |
| **Mental Health** | | |
| Ever received mental health treatment*** | 2.039 | (1.484, 2.800) |
| **Criminal Justice** | | |
| Reported receiving criminal justice services at any admission(b)*** | 1.892 | (1.427, 2.510) |
| **Drug Treatment** | | |
| Mean number of treatments*** | 1.093 | (1.065, 1.122) |
| **Drug Use** | | |
| Reported injecting drugs in the month prior to last intake*** | .407 | (.305, .544) |

Model Chi Square $\chi^2 = 610.599$, df = 15, $p < .000$
Nagelkerke R Square = .409
(a) Reference group
(b) Yes group is compared to the no group
* $p \leq .05$, ** $p \leq .01$, *** $p \leq .001$.

methadone treatment. Yet, health insurance status was not associated with use of residential treatment. These patterns are likely explained by funding sources for treatment in Massachusetts. For example, many residential programs receive funding from the state health department and might be less dependent on health insurance coverage.

Second, involvement in the mental health and criminal justice systems was especially associated with an increase in the likelihood of receiving residential treatment, as was the number of previous entries into substance abuse treatment. Given that residential treatment programs provide the most comprehensive system of services, compared to detoxification and methadone maintenance, it is encouraging to find that the Hispanic women who need these services the most–those with mental health histories–also entered this type of treatment. On the other hand, this finding points to the possibility that women drug users linked to other service systems, here mental health and criminal justice, were the most likely to receive the most comprehensive drug treatment services, possibly as a result of mandated treatment referrals. A recent study by Amaro and colleagues (Amaro, Larson, Gampel, Richardson, Savage, & Wagler, in press) found that compared to Black and White women in treatment, Hispanic women were significantly more likely to be mandated to treatment and to have recent jail experience. Thus, among Hispanic women, criminal justice involvement seems to be an enabling factor for entering residential treatment. Further, the findings also highlight that co-occurring mental disorders among Hispanic women in substance abuse treatment play an important role in access to treatment and that substance abuse treatment services need to integrate treatment for mental health problems (Amaro, Nieves, Wolde Johannes, & Labault Cabeza, 1999; Amaro et al., in press).

Third, the analysis also identified that there were significant differences in types of drug treatment entered by Hispanic women. Specifically, Puerto Rican women were significantly more likely to enter methadone maintenance and significantly less likely to enter only detoxification. This difference was especially pronounced with respect to methadone maintenance with Puerto Rican women being more than one and a half times more likely to enter this treatment modality compared to other Hispanic women.

A fourth and final pattern which emerged is similar to a finding from another study (Lundgren, Schilling, Ferguson, Davis, & Amodeo, 2003) which shows that human capital factors such as employment, health insurance, and parental status are associated with type of treatment entered. Hence, those with no insurance, who are not working, who do not have children or no longer reside with their children are most likely to have entered only detoxification. Whereas detoxification provides critically needed services–it is a pre-drug-treatment modality–individuals who use only detoxification are probably less likely to change drug use behaviors compared to those who use methadone maintenance and residential treatment. Further, multiple use of detoxification evidences continual high level use of drugs.

What then are the social work practice implications of these findings? First, these findings would suggest that social work practitioners working with Hispanic women IDUs need to more actively promote the use of residential treatment services to this group, especially those not yet involved with the mental health and criminal justice systems. Previous research (Lundgren et al., 2003) indicates that overall, Hispanics are less likely than other groups to use residential treatment programs. Similarly, research in mental health (U.S. Department of Health and Human Services, 1999), substance abuse (Arroyo, Miller, & Tonigan, 2003; Weiss, Kung, & Pearson, 2003), and medical care (Smedley, Stith, & Nelson, 2003) indicates that racial and ethnic differences are important factors to consider in the design of services.

The current study suggests that those Hispanic women who do receive residential treatment do this as a result of having been part of other service systems, specifically mental health and criminal justice systems. Therefore strong linkages between substance abuse treatment services and the mental health care delivery system and the criminal justice system may be especially important avenues to facilitate referral and use of residential treatment among Hispanic women. In addition, because Hispanic women who enter residential treatment and methadone treatment may be more likely to have co-occurring mental health problems, social workers who work in residential treatment programs with Hispanic women should receive specialized training on the treatment of co-occurring mental health and addiction disorders.

Also, social work practitioners need to be aware that different groups of Hispanic women either prefer or are referred to different types of treatment services. In this study, Puerto Rican women compared to other groups of Hispanic women were significantly more likely to use methadone maintenance. It is beyond the scope of this study to identify whether or not these patterns of treatment used are the result of either client preference or specific referral procedures.

There is a dearth of scientific literature on drug treatment utilization among various groups of Hispanic women and little information is available to assess whether the differences between Puerto Rican and other Hispanic women observed in this study are related to differences in knowledge about the various treatment modalities, attitudes toward these modalities of treatment, or systemic barriers to such programs.

## *LIMITATIONS*

The findings of this study should be considered in light of the following limitations: First, the data set used does not capture treatment the IDUs may have received before 1996 or after 2002; individuals may have been at the beginning or end of a treatment career that lasted more than the seven years reported here. Nonetheless, over seven years, many IDUs will enter and complete treatment, experience some abstinence or reduced use, relapse for some weeks or months, often repeatedly experience the common cycle of abstinence or less harmful use, relapse, and treatment reentry. Second, only "formal" drug treatments were examined, and thus the study did not consider 12-step meetings or private psychotherapy. Third, as the data are from Massachusetts only, future studies should include comparisons across multiple states. Fourth, the data were obtained via intake interviews conducted by a diverse group of staff from many treatment settings. Finally, the sample of non-Puerto Rican Hispanic women was too small to allow us to investigate differences in patterns of treatment entry among subgroups categorized under Other Hispanics.

## REFERENCES

Aday, L., & Awe, C. (1997). Health services utilization models. In D. S. Gochman (Ed.), *Handbook of Health Behavior Research 1: Personal and Social Determinants.* New York and London: Plenum Press.

Amaro, H., Nieves, R., Wolde Johannes, S., & Labault Cabeza, N. (1999). Substance abuse treatment: Critical issues and challenges in the treatment of Latina women. *Hispanic Journal of Behavioral Sciences*, 21(3), 266-282.

Amaro, H., Larson, M.J., Gampel, J., Richardson, E., Savage, A., & Wagler, D. (in press). Racial/Ethnic Differences in Social Vulnerability among Women with Co-occurring Mental Health and Substance Abuse Disorders: Implications for Treatment Services. *Journal of Community Psychology.*

Amaro, H., Whitaker, R., Coffman, G. & Heeren, T. (1990). Acculturation and marijuana and cocaine use: Findings from the Hispanic HANES. *American Journal of Public Health*, 80, pp. 54-60.

Andersen, R. (1995). Revisiting the behavioral model and access to medical care: Does it matter? *Journal of Health and Social Behavior,* 36, pp. 1-10.

Arroyo, J.A., Miller, W.R., & Tonigan, J.S. (2003). The influence of Hispanic ethnicity on long-term outcome in three alcohol treatment modalities. *Journal of Studies on Alcohol*, 64(1), 98-104.

Centers for Disease Control and Prevention. (2002). *HIV/AIDS surveillance report 2002*; 14:1-148. Retrieved April 2, 2004 from: http://www.cdc.gov/hiv/stats/hasrlink.htm.

COSSMHO (National Coalition of Hispanic Health and Human Service Organizations). (1991). HIV/AIDS–The impact on Hispanics in selected states. Washington, DC: COSSMHO.

Diaz, T., Buehler, J.W., Castro, K.G., & Ward, J.W. (1993). AIDS trends among Hispanics in the United States. *American Journal of Public Health,* 83, pp. 504-509.

Frank, B. (2000). An overview of heroin trends in New York City: Past, present, and future. *Mount Sinai Journal of Medicine*, 67(5-6), pp. 340-6.

Hser, Y., Grella, C., Shih-Chao, H., Anglin, M.D., & Brown, B. (1999). Prior treatment experience related to process and outcomes in DATOS. *Drug and Alcohol Dependence*, 57, pp. 137-150.

Kaiser Family Foundation. (2002). *State health facts on-line. Massachusetts: Cumulative AIDS cases by exposure category, reported through December 2001*. Retrieved April 2, 2004 from: http://www.statehealthfacts.kff.org/cgi-bin/healthfacts.cgi?action=profile&area=Massachusetts&welcome=1&category=HIV%2fAIDS.

Lundgren, L., Amodeo, M., Ferguson, F., & Davis, K. (2001). Racial and ethnic difference in drug treatment entry of injection drug users in Massachusetts. *Journal of Substance Abuse Treatment*, 2, pp. 145-153.

Lundgren, L., & Ben-Ami, L. (2004) Patterns of drug-treatment entry, Massachusetts, 1996-2002. Unpublished Report, Boston University. Boston, MA.

Lundgren, L., Schilling, R., Ferguson, F., Davis, K., & Amodeo, M. (2003). Examining drug treatment program entry of injection drug users: Human capital and institutional disaffiliation. *Evaluation and Program Planning*, 26, pp.123-132.

Massachusetts Department of Public Health, Bureau of Substance Abuse Services. (2003). *Substance abuse fact sheet: Adult women admissions, 2003*. Retrieved April 2, 2004 from: http://www.state.ma.us/dph/bsas/data/factsheets/2002/Women02 Final_.doc

McCarty, D., McGuire, T.G., Harwood, H.J., & Field, T. (1998). Using state information systems for drug abuse services research. *American Behavioral Scientist*, 41(8), pp. 1090-1106.

National Institute on Drug Abuse (NIDA). (1992). Data from the National AIDS Demonstrations Research Program (NADR). Rockville, MD: National Institute on Drug Abuse.

Robles, RR., Matos, T.D., Colon, H.M., Deren, S., Reyes, J.C., Andia, J., Marrero, C.A., & Sahai, H. (2003). Determinants of health care use among Puerto Rican drug users in Puerto Rico and New York City. *Clinical Infectious Diseases*, 37, Suppl 5, pp. S392-403.

Selik, R.M., Castro, K.G., & Pappaioanou, M. (1989). Birthplace and the risk for AIDS among Hispanics in the United States. *American Journal of Public Health*, 79, pp. 836-839.

Selik, R.M., Castro, K.G., & Pappaioanou, M. (1988). Racial/ethnic differences in the risk of AIDS in the United States. *American Journal of Public Health*, 78, pp. 1539-1545.

Smedley, B.D., Stith, A.Y., & Nelson, A.R. (2003). *Unequal treatment: Confronting racial and ethnic disparities in health care.* Washington, DC: National Academy Press.

Substance Abuse and Mental Health Services Administration. (SAMHSA). (2002a). Results from the 2001 National Household Survey on Drug Abuse: Volume I. summary of national findings. Office of Applied Studies, NHSDA Series H-17, DHHS Publications No. SMA 02-3758. Rockville, MD.

Substance Abuse and Mental Health Services Administration (SAMHSA). (2002b). Hispanics in substance abuse treatment: 1999. Drug and Alcohol Services Information System Report, September 2, 2002. Rockville, MD: Office of Applied Studies, SAMHSA.

Substance Abuse and Mental Health Services Administration. (2003a). *Emergency department trends from the Drug Abuse Warning Network, Final Estimates 1995-2002*, August 2003. Retrieved April 2, 2004 from: http//:dawninfo.samhsa.gov/ pubs_94_02/ edpubs/2002final/.

Substance Abuse and Mental Health Services Administration. (SAMHSA). (2003b).Overview of findings from the 2002 National Survey on Drug Use and Health (Office of Applied Studies, NHSDA Series H-21, DHHS Publication No. SMA03-3774). Rockville, MD.

U. S. Department of Health and Human Services. (1999). Mental health: Culture, race, ethnicity-Supplement. Rockville, MD: U.S. Department of Health and Human Services, Substance Abuse and Services Administration, Center for Mental Health Services, National Institutes of Health, National Institute of Mental Health.

U. S. Bureau of the Census. (2000). Retrieved August 15, 2003 from http://www.census.gov.

Weiss, S.R., Kung, H.C., & Pearson, J.L. (2003). Emerging issues in gender and ethnic differences in substance abuse and treatment. *Current Women's Health Reports*, 3(3), 245-253.

# SPECIAL TOPICS

# HIV/AIDS Prevention Practice with Latino/a Substance Abusers: An Interview with Jennifer Herrera

This interview was conducted by Lori K. Holleran

*Holleran*: As Director of Prevention Programs, AIDS Services of Austin, Texas, how do you perceive substance abuse issues as they relate to Latinos/as that you encounter in your work? Who is effected and how?

*Herrera*: We know that poverty has a huge impact on the Latino community and that addiction, many times, is not the problem, but rather the result or coping mechanism by which people deal with life stressors. In our work we have seen a strong correlation between individuals who are

Jennifer Herrera, BA, is Director of Prevention Services, AIDS Services in Austin, and has worked in AIDS services for almost five years. Lori K. Holleran, PhD, was an Addictions Therapist and worked in prevention. Currently, she is Assistant Professor, University of Texas, Austin, focusing on the area of Mexican American youth and culturally grounded drug prevention. She has recently received a 5-year K01 Mentored Research Scientist Award from NIH.

[Haworth co-indexing entry note]: "HIV/AIDS Prevention Practice with Latino/a Substance Abusers: An Interview with Jennifer Herrera." Holleran, Lori K. Co-published simultaneously in *Journal of Social Work Practice in the Addictions* (The Haworth Press, Inc.) Vol. 5, No. 1/2, 2005, pp. 175-183; and: *Substance Abusing Latinos: Current Research on Epidemiology, Prevention, and Treatment* (ed: Mario R. De La Rosa, Lori K. Holleran, and Shulamith Lala Ashenberg Straussner) The Haworth Press, Inc., 2005, pp. 175-183. Single or multiple copies of this article are available for a fee from The Haworth Document Delivery Service [1-800-HAWORTH, 9:00 a.m. - 5:00 p.m. (EST). E-mail address: docdelivery@haworthpress.com].

http://www.haworthpress.com/web/JSWPA

Digital Object Identifier: 10.1300/J160v05n01_09

undocumented, uninsured, impoverished, dealing with undiagnosed mental health issues and isolated as the main factors contributing to substance abuse and addiction. Latino men who are out of work and unable to provide for their families (in the U.S., in Mexico, or in both places) many times will express their feelings of failure and indicate that this is why they start to use alcohol and/or other drugs excessively. Over the past 3 years we have seen an increase in the number of men that will self-report that they are injecting heroin or smoking crack. Many men also describe that they occasional use spray paints and glues because they are easily accessible through their work sites.

We find that Latina women are much less likely to disclose substance abuse issues. We have had women share their experiences with alcohol and occasionally crack-cocaine, but most often their risk factors for HIV are due to multiple sex partners or the risk factors of their sexual partners. Our work has shown us that since Latina women are often the caretakers for their children they are very resistant to sharing information about their drug use or abuse because they fear that their children will be taken away.

*Holleran*: What unique and emerging issues exist for these individuals and what are your biggest concerns and challenges in relation to these issues?

*Herrera*: The most challenging issues we continue to see throughout the Latino community involves the dependency of Latina women on Latino men. Many of the Latina women we work with are from Mexico and South America and have limited education. Many are illiterate and most often they have multiple children to care for. These women are undocumented and rely solely, or very heavily, on the men's income to provide for their families. Confronting their partner's behaviors such as alcohol or other drug use increases the risk of losing that income that maintains the basic needs of the family. Such power dynamics also mean that many women continue to remain with a violent and abusive partner for fear of losing that person's financial support. These women often have feelings of depression, helplessness and isolation because they know that their partners may be abusing substances and/or having sex with multiple partners outside of their relationship, but they cannot, or will not, confront them out of fear and shame.

In our work with men at various day labor sites, another issue that continues to arise is the number of men from Mexico or South America that have left their country of origin in search of a better future financially and/or to escape persecution because they are gay. We have been amazed at the number of men who have openly disclosed that they are having sex with men, and self-identify as gay. These men have often left families that had abandoned or "disowned" them because of their sexual orientation, leaving the men feeling completely cut off from their support systems and very isolated. They are usually willing to disclose this to our peer educators but are not willing to share this information with the entire group. We continue to see the prevalence of drug use among these men due to issues of shame and guilt. Furthermore, many men have shared with us that they are only able to have sex with other men if alcohol or other substances are involved. Being intoxicated or under the influence helps "justify" sexual behaviors that they consider "inappropriate" or "morally wrong."

*Holleran*: Can you provide some anecdotes that illustrate substance abuse scenarios among the Latino/a clients or others that are touched by your preventionists at AIDS Services of Austin (ASA)?

*Herrera*: We recently met a Latino male who is actively using heroin, HIV positive, and in search of both treatment and medical services. This person had only been in Texas a few months, but was aware of his HIV status and has been in and out of drug treatment programs throughout the years. He had learned about our work and our services through a "friend on the streets" and contacted ASA. We called our partnering agency at the MHMR (Mental Health and Mental Retardation) CARE (Community AIDS Resource Education) Drop-In-Center and both our prevention staff member along with a staff person from CARE (who specialize in substance abuse and HIV) met the client at the Salvation Army. After setting up an intake appointment for him at CARE and a medical appointment at our medical facility, our team got the necessary paperwork filled out to provide him with temporary housing until his intake appointment at CARE. The client was also given food so that he would not have to wait in "soup kitchen" lines while feeling ill. Without this assistance the client would have stayed on the streets and may have remained out of medical care. In meeting him, our team also gained his trust, so much so, that he let us see his abscess and determine if it was in need of immediate medical care. Having two skilled workers (one with a 15-year heroin addiction and clean another 20 years) gave us the expertise we needed to reassure him that the wound was not infected and to show how to properly clean it so it did not get infected. The client is on a waiting list for an in-patient drug treatment program.

Another client is a Latino male with alcohol addiction and Hepatitis C. He was experiencing great pain and discomfort due to his liver problems. This client approached us during our presentation at a day labor site. We were able to meet with the client privately, give him information about Hep C and educate him about the correlation between his liver problems and alcohol consumption. While complete abstinence was not an option for him at this stage, he now has a better understanding of the link between the two and has tried to cut down his alcohol intake. He was also taking Tylenol for his body aches and pains; we also provided him with information about the dangers of this drug for people living with Hep C. Previously, he had visited a public clinic and was sent away with a Hep C brochure in English, which he couldn't read, and some pills (he had no idea what he was given). Although there was not much more we could do for him, due to limited medical services available for Spanish speaking people with Hep C, he was extremely grateful and has since introduced us to another three individuals living with Hep C so that we could provide them with some information.

In an effort to better reach our highest risk clients, we purposefully stopped going to the day labor site at 4 a.m. and decided to move the time to 8 a.m. Our theory was that men who are healthy and not using substances are more likely to find jobs and be at work at 4 a.m. Those that show up later in the morning are often older, not physically well, have stayed out "partying" the night before, and may also be dealing with substance abuse issues. So far, our theory and strategy has proven to be effective. We are seeing a larger number of men who are dealing with substance related issues and who are seeking additional information or referrals to drug treatment programs after listening to our workshops.

Three years ago, we started to provide outreach services to Latina women in low-income apartment complexes in Austin. Initially, after discouraging outcomes and realizing that the women would not engage in conversations with us because they were fearful about what we were there to do, we decided to take another approach. Having two Latina women on our prevention team gave us the insight that the women would not talk with us until we had an established "gatekeeper." A gatekeeper is someone from within the community that is able to make firsthand introductions and has established a trusting relationship with the community being targeted. Our next strategy was to work with the men at the nearby day labor site, develop rapport, build trust and then gain their permission to meet their sexual partners who lived in the nearby apartments. Almost two years later, our strategy proved to be effective and we were not only successful in having the men link us to their female partners, but the female partners then helped us to recruit their female family members, friends and neighbors.

As of July 2004, we have conducted over a dozen "platicas" (talks) with the Latina women from the neighborhoods close to the day labor sites. These platicas have consisted of basic facts about HIV; myths; cultural factors contributing to lack of testing and risk reduction; reproductive health; condom negotiation; benefits to using condoms; learning about condom features; harm reduction/risk reduction strategies; substance use/abuse; communication skills; body mapping and self-esteem. These workshops begin as a one-hour small group session and then advance to 3-hour sessions. During the sessions the women explore their feelings about risk reduction, learn and practice skills to reduce their risk factors, and become more aware about the connection between risk reduction and protecting or maintaining their own wellness. Groups are a mixture of psycho-educational information, empathic support, skill practice (e.g., using condoms, articulating needs, etc.), and processing feelings.

*Holleran*: I know that the ASA Prevention Team does some fabulous, innovative work with Latinos/as. Can you describe some of the interventions and perhaps what you have witnessed (both positive and negative) in response?

*Herrera*: I will try and describe what our interventions look like in practice:

- Our peer educators, who are indigenous to the communities we serve, rely on their knowledge and familiarity with the neighborhoods to help us identify areas we consider to be high-risk. These areas often consist of congregations of Latinas/os who are living in poverty, the working poor who are uninsured, have a higher prevalence to drug addition, or drug trafficking, multiple children, high rates of sex work (sex for money, drugs or survival), and according to local HIV/STD data, places with higher incidences of people living with STD infections.
- Experienced peer educators enter these communities trained in delivering effective outreach providing information, referrals and risk reduction kits (condoms, water-based lube and testing info). Peer educators stop people who are walking on the streets, at day labor sites, Laundromats, parking lots, stores, apartment com-

plexes, gas stations, liquor stores, and parks. During these encounters they introduce themselves, the agency and what they are attempting to do. Each client is told that our goal is to raise awareness throughout our Latino communities about the importance of HIV information, testing and services for people living with the disease. The teams are always treated with great respect and have earned the trust of the community.

- The constant presence and trust established has earned the staff the ability to not just meet the community members, but they are invited into the community members' "lives" through their shared stories and experiences. The community members have shared their risk factors past and present and have helped our staff by introducing us to their families and friends. A few key members have introduced us to their sexual partners and those partners have then introduced us to their network of family and friends.
- This "ripple" effect helped us to recruit for our very first "platica" (talk) with Latinas interested in learning more about what we are doing. The first informal talk was scheduled at the agency located close by one of the targeted apartment complexes. Handwritten invitations were delivered to over 15 women and followed by continued outreach visits reminding them about the event. The first event attracted 12 women.
- The 12 women were invited to a 1-hour platica hosted by two peer educators. These staff facilitated the entire workshop in Spanish. Mexican food was purchased for the participants from a local Latina taco shop owner. The food was spicy and the topics too. The women started off with an icebreaker in which the facilitators shared a secret with one woman and that woman was asked to whisper the secret to her neighbor. The secret was passed among the entire group and the last woman was asked to share her secret. The end result showed how dramatically different the last secret was from the first. The facilitators then tied this back to how HIV information is shared and spread throughout our community. How quickly misinformation can be passed and how that misinformation can be harmful and possibly "hurtful." Ground rules for the discussion are agreed upon, then the women are asked this question: Why don't Latinas access HIV prevention services and HIV testing? The women are given a few examples and then asked to contribute to the list. Some initial comments are made, such as fear of deportation, or fear of someone finding out. The women are asked to share and process these factors. The women are then

asked to share and to discuss "What are benefits to accessing HIV prevention services and testing?"

- These findings allow our staff to access meaningful information about factors that may be influencing the women's willingness to participate in future prevention programs. For example, many women said that "childcare" was one of the biggest factors influencing their ability to access care. This allowed us to explore options or solutions for dealing with this obstacle. As a result, when ASA hosted our next event we had both staff and volunteers help take care of the children while the mothers participated in the intervention. The children were encouraged to color, play with blocks, puzzles, and puppets, providing them with an opportunity to express themselves through activities and not just sit in front of a television.
- The women attending these platicas are also asked at the end of the session to tell us what they enjoyed about the discussion and what other topics they would like to explore.
- Two weeks later, these same women are then invited to bring guests and attend VOICES/VOCES. VOCES is a 60-minute single-session small group Effective Behavioral Intervention program, proven through research to have an impact on risk reduction behaviors. The program consists of viewing a culturally specific video, building condom negotiation skills, providing information about different types of condoms and distributing condom samples. Food and child care along with incentives such as bubble baths, gels, relaxation beads and hair accessories are given as prizes for attending.
- Two weeks later, the women are invited to bring a guest to a two-hour platica on the female reproductive system, basic female anatomy, body mapping and self-esteem. First the women are given a printed diagram of the female reproductive system along with a brief description about what each "part" is and how it works, then using Play Dough the women are instructed to create their own vaginas including the cervix, uterus, fallopian tubes and uterus. During their creations the facilitators answer questions about menstruation, ovulation, pregnancy and STD's. Next, the women are given newsprint and they are instructed to draw themselves indicating all the parts of their bodies they "love." They are then invited to share with the group their drawings. This allows the women to share and explore their self-body image, feelings about

their sexuality, and to affirm their positive feelings and explore their negative feelings about themselves.

- After this activity the women are invited to lay down on pillows, lights dimmed, and listen to relaxing music. The facilitator takes them through a breathing relaxation activity and then expresses lots of affirmations about their value, importance, beauty and uniqueness.
- These women are then invited back to a longer intervention (RARA) Reducing AIDS Risk Activities. RARA is designed to assist Latina women in developing and maintaining a sound sexual health plan. This program consists of four (1 1/2 to 2 hour) meetings including videotape stimulus. The program encourages women to think about the physical and emotional consequences of unsafe sex. It helps them achieve a sense of mastery and develop positive expectations when performing a wide variety of behaviors related to sexual health, including talking about sexual history with partners, HIV testing, plans for monogamy, condom use, refusal of alcohol and drugs, and general assertiveness training. Again, food, childcare and incentives are provided during each of these sessions.

*Holleran*: I know that you work from an ecological and transtheoretical base. Can you elaborate on your conceptual foundations and the evidence-based interventions that you utilize with Latino/a substance abusers?

*Herrera*: It has been our experience that outreach allows for our staff to plant the "seeds" of thought to people throughout the community about how substance abuse and HIV may or may not be affecting them. This outreach concept really allows for the opportunity to introduce ambivalence to those persons who may be either in a precontemplative or contemplative state of change regarding HIV, substance abuse and risk reduction. The interventions, workshops, and platicas serve to reach those that may be more in a contemplative or readiness state of change but lack the information, skills for change, or are feeling unsure about what and how those changes may affect their lives.

Many of the interventions work at providing the tools necessary to help someone help themselves in discovering what types of changes they are ready and able to make, how to go about making those changes, and what may be some of the consequences to changing. These interventions may also serve to promote continued change for those who have made reductions in their risk taking, but are in need of validation and encouragement while maintaining those actions. All of our prevention efforts center around a Harm Reduction model, understanding that people change their behaviors when they are ready, wanting, and able to change, and that our services must address the clients' changing and diverse needs and not our own agendas.

*Holleran*: What are your recommendations (i.e., "words of wisdom" or skills for a practical "bag of tricks") for social workers and others who work or may want to work clinically with this population? Also, are there any specific resources that you would recommend such clinicians to access?

*Herrera*: The community members have the answers to the questions we as providers are constantly seeking. Ask them what they want to know, how they feel, who this is affecting, why it matters, when they want our services and how those services need to be delivered. Reaching the Latino community means identifying what matters most to the individuals you are trying to reach. If it means caring for their families, then find the link that shows them that taking care of themselves means caring for their families. If providing for their families is most important, then show them how taking care of themselves means they will be well enough and fit enough to do just that. We have to approach people where "they are at" and find out what matters most to them, honor that, and understand that while HIV or addiction may not be their top priority, respect their process and understand that sometimes our roles can just be to listen and find out what our clients are most concerned about. That process and our willingness to listen echoes deep within our clients' hearts and when they are ready to address issues that are on OUR agenda, they will know who they can turn to for support and services and that we will provide those services with compassion and care.

*Holleran*: Your expertise, empathy, and experience are deeply appreciated. Would you be willing to have journal readers contact you if they have questions or comments?

*Herrera*: Yes, by all means. I can be reached by e-mail at: jennifer.herrera@asaustin.org

# The Story of a Bi-Cultural, Latina Addict

Evelyn B.

I am a First Generation American. My mother was from Mexico of Spanish and German descent and my father was from British Honduras (now Belize) of British and Spanish decent. Both of my parents were raised with a strong Hispanic Catholic foundation. We spoke only Spanish at home. English was what we learned in school. I vacationed with my seven siblings, maternal grandmother, and Mayan nannies every summer for three months on the beach in the Yucatan Peninsula. There we lived in a large thatched roof home, slept in hammocks, walked two blocks to gather water from the drinking well (baths were salt water) and of course no electricity. In Yucatan we were announced in the local papers, "the Gringas have arrived!"

Back home in the U.S., our classmates and friends felt we were unique because we spoke Spanish, had relatives in Mexico, and for

Evelyn B., a single mother of a 4-year-old son, lives and works in a small town in Texas. She has been sober for five years. She continues to work the 12-Step principals of AA and spends her free time helping other women alcoholics and alcoholic family members.

[Haworth co-indexing entry note]: "The Story of a Bi-Cultural, Latina Addict." B., Evelyn. Co-published simultaneously in *Journal of Social Work Practice in the Addictions* (The Haworth Press, Inc.) Vol. 5, No. 1/2, 2005, pp. 185-189; and: *Substance Abusing Latinos: Current Research on Epidemiology, Prevention, and Treatment* (ed: Mario R. De La Rosa, Lori K. Holleran, and Shulamith Lala Ashenberg Straussner) The Haworth Press, Inc., 2005, pp. 185-189. Single or multiple copies of this article are available for a fee from The Haworth Document Delivery Service [1-800-HAWORTH, 9:00 a.m. - 5:00 p.m. (EST). E-mail address: docdelivery@haworthpress.com].

http://www.haworthpress.com/web/JSWPA

Digital Object identifier: 10.1300/J160v05n01_10

breakfast we ate scrambled eggs, refried beans, and hand made tortillas, an atypical breakfast in New Orleans, Louisiana.

I remember that I wanted to belong so badly; I concluded early on that I didn't fit anywhere. As soon as I could, I left home. However, due to my parents' beliefs, the only way that I could leave was to be married. The Church simply did not condone daughters leaving their families on their own. Just barely 18 years old, threatening to elope, my parents gave me away to a young man they knew was not for me.

I married Jorge and within two months of our marriage he began beating me when he drank. I kept this horrible secret from my family. After eight months of physical abuse, I told my parents the truth; they responded, "You made your bed; now lie in it."

I went to one of Jorge's friends for help and he suggested that I smoke marijuana. He said I would feel much better about the situation. I tried marijuana and loved it. I used alcohol when I could not smoke marijuana. Finally, with the help of marijuana and alcohol, I found the courage to leave Jorge and did not care what others thought. I was considered a disgrace to the family name. My separation was kept from the rest of my relatives. I could only imagine their reaction to my drinking and using drugs. I suspected they would disown me if they ever found out.

My secret grew; I was drinking, smoking marijuana, and ingesting just about any drug I was offered. I thought that I was still in control. At the same time, I had the deep, insidious feeling that I was "no good" and that no one would ever want me. I dated several men and became promiscuous. One day, on a weekend vacation in Cancun, I met my future husband. Manolo was a very wealthy businessman from Mexico City. He was ten years my senior. I remember asking him if he wanted to share some "fine marijuana." He told me that he despised drugs. Feeling ashamed, I offered him bottles of wine. We began drinking together.

Three months after we met, Manolo invited me on a trip to Spain. Spain was wonderful. We drank wine all day and all night. Upon returning from our trip, Manolo proposed to me. My parents were elated that their divorced daughter was worthy of marrying a powerful and wealthy man like Manolo. However, my best friend did point out to me that Manolo was a heavy drinker. I told her, "Never you mind; at least he doesn't beat me."

We went on a European and Mediterranean honeymoon. I was surprised at my new and wonderful life. I did not use drugs anymore; I felt that the fancy champagne was more appropriate for an individual of my "new stature" anyway. Life changed dramatically for me. My friends in the USA no longer understood my lifestyle. Eventually, I lost all contact with them. I didn't have any friends in Mexico City the first three years there either. I would awaken at 1:00 p.m., get dressed and meet my husband for lunch at 2:00. These lunches were often with people that I did not particularly care for. They were either my husband's colleagues or business clients. "Lunch" was not over until 1:00 or 2:00 a.m.

After a while, I became keenly aware that my husband was an alcoholic. Certainly I wasn't an alcoholic, I thought, because he drank far more than I and he was the one who acted inappropriately. I became depressed. I could not tell my parents how my life really was. How would this look, a second marriage gone wrong? My husband was so charming and my parents loved him. In their eyes he could do no wrong. Manolo gave me all and anything I desired. I would be foolish to leave a man of such socio-economic standing.

Manolo had two types of friends: his associates, who were people who had literally succeeded in the business world from the bottom up, and the "Old Rich" (this group included his family). I felt superior to some and inferior to others, but did not feel like a peer to anyone. I felt I had to keep switching personalities to impress and please my husband. Despite my family roots in Mexico, I was still not acknowledged as part of that culture. In the U.S., I was not an American either. I did not feel connected to either place. I stood between cultures, desperate to belong.

After eight years of living lies and deceit, a friend suggested that I attend Al-Anon for family members of addicts/alcoholics. She said that there were people there who felt as I did and they could help me if I wanted. At my first meeting, I did not feel understood because I was an American and my Spanish was awful. I believed that they did not understand me because of my Latina-Anglo experience. However, I now realize that I often have used my bi-cultural identity as a crutch, an excuse to continue to relieve myself with substances and perpetuate my self-pity. I did stop drinking during my early recovery in Al-Anon. I learned a new way of life and had completely different thoughts about who I was and what my purpose in life was. I became less sensitive to being called a "Gringa," and I didn't feel compelled any longer to explain that I was also Latina. I found myself fitting in with others in 12-Step programs because of our common feelings and experiences. In my ninth year in Al-Anon, I was active in service and it was wonderful. While helping others, it did not matter what ethnicity I was. I felt I had "recovered."

I started to see an Acupuncturist for infertility. I had tried for 13 years to conceive with no success. I was told that this man, Javier, could help me and I had already tried all the conventional medical procedures. I began to have deep feelings for him. One day, he mentioned to me that one of his patient's didn't have money to pay him so he had given him as payment a small amount of cocaine. I convinced him that we should use it together and my alcoholic progression took off once again.

I had an affair; alcohol and cocaine gave me courage to live this lifestyle. My life became a lie. As time went by, I considered divorcing my husband. In my mind I rationalized that I could continue my relationship with Javier, and alcohol and drugs.

One day I realized that everything we owned was in my husband's name only. He always used the excuse that an American could not own any property in Mexico and I believed him. We had been married for 14 years and he didn't have a will in place in case something happened to him. I decided to investigate all the paperwork that he asked me to sign during our marriage. (When I would ask, "What is this?" he would reply, "Just do as I say; it's for us." My mother raised me to never question my husband's authority, so I just signed away.) It became clear that my husband had done many things without my knowing, some even illegal. My husband never said anything to me even when I would try to bring it up. I was advised by my lawyers to leave the country. Where was I to go? What was I to do? I knew that I had a serious problem with addiction and was I was very fearful.

God had never abandoned me, so I took my faith, my little dog, and automobile and drove a straight line out of Mexico City into Texas. I rented an apartment and spent many days in that apartment, drinking. In my mind, Americans could not possibly understand my predicament. They just didn't understand what I knew about my culture–the shame of leaving my husband; the shame of being a drug addicted alcoholic woman.

I decided to get sober and went to my first Alcoholics Anonymous meeting. I remember whining about missing my homes, trips, cars, and opulent lifestyle. Everyone laughed. In time, I began to come out of the fog I was in. I began to go out with people in the program and I remember still being a bit reserved because I still didn't feel like I belonged. My Latin culture seemed to get in the way.

My sponsor did not seem to be concerned with the culture differences when I would mention this to her. She only found them interesting, not controversial or detrimental to my recovery. I certainly was full of self-pity. What was I to do? My sponsor always answered this question by responding, "Work the 12 steps of Alcoholics Anonymous." Here are a few things I learned in AA:

- I am not unique. I have learned that all Alcoholics believe they are different. It is part of the disease.
- I don't have to blame my bi-cultural upbringing for my feelings of not belonging.
- I use rationalizations in order to justify my actions.
- It doesn't matter where I came from. Alcohol doesn't discriminate.
- I used my bi-cultural upbringing as a crutch so as not to belong, neither here nor there. In AA, it falls under the category of self-centeredness and isolation.
- I had a big part in what happened to me in my life.
- I have power to change myself and choose my actions.
- I am no longer dependent on what my family believes is right or wrong.

I no longer consider myself an outsider in the world. I believe that I have been given an opportunity to have multiple experiences and that these experiences serve me to help others. My bi-cultural background today is absolutely a gift. What better place than in United States to have such knowledge about different peoples and their customs, traditions, and lifestyles.

This is my message to other bi-cultural women that are feeling stuck in old tradition from another culture. Here, as women, we have a choice. Either continue to be the submissive individual and continue to wallow in self-pity or exercise our God-given right to be anything we want.

# Index



 

9780789028822